This book is due for return on or b

ATLAS OF ENVIRONMENTAL DERMATOLOGY

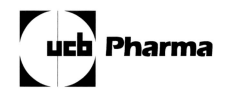

Dépôt Légal : D/1997/5.541-8
ISBN : 2-87301-022-3
© UCB Pharma Sector - Braine-l'Alleud - Belgium 1994

Responsible Editor :	Diane VAN MOERBEKE
	Chemin du Foriest
	B-1420 Braine-l'Alleud - Belgium
Lay-out :	Dino Drusi Communication
Printing :	Imprimerie Cartiaux-Pierard

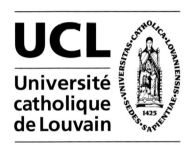

UCL
Université
catholique
de Louvain

Jean-Marie **LACHAPELLE**
Professor in Dermatology,
University Hospital Saint-Luc, UCL Brussels
and University Hospital Mont-Godinne

Dominique **TENNSTEDT**
Consultant,
University Hospital Saint-Luc,
UCL Brussels

Liliane **MAROT**
External consultant,
University Hospital Mont-Godinne,
UCL Yvoir

CONTENTS

FOREWORD

The Atlas of Environmental Dermatology complements the Atlas of General Dermatology published in 1994. Of the array of such atlases published worldwide, some are intended to introduce non specialists to common skin lesions in general practice. Others are aimed at a particular field within the specialty : pediatric, geriatric or pregnancy dermatology, for example, or the dermatology of particular skin regions (topographic dermatology) or skin types (dermatology of black skin). Even more focussed atlases are those addressing specific conditions : viral and bacterial dermatoses, mycoses, drug eruptions, tropical dermatoses, sexually transmitted dermatoses etc.

It was our conviction that this profusion could only be further enriched by an Atlas of Environmental Dermatology. Today's environment has undergone such changes that it has either engendered new diseases or modified the presentation of familiar dermatoses.

Two years have passed since that original inspiration. The Atlas is internationalist in outlook and is thus virtually entirely devoted to cosmopolitan dermatoses. This has involved incorporating a few dermatoses that are imported into temperate zones, such as *larva migrans*. Exclusively tropical dermatoses feature only exceptionally, e.g. Buruli ulcer, for the purpose of comparison with cosmopolitan mycobacterioses or South American leishmaniasis. Most illustrations show conditions encountered on white skin, but some environmental dermatoses largely specific to black skin are included in the different sections of the Atlas.

The problem of classification was the subject of many hours thought. Despite – or perhaps because of – a concern for maximum rigour, the "ideal" classification has not been achieved : any attempt at classification is likely to invite constructive criticism from the expert reader.

Sexually transmitted diseases, including those related to AIDS, have been deliberately omitted.

The major challenge of the 21st century is to prevent all environmental dermatoses and develop effective therapy for those that still occur. In terms of prevention, the table presented by Klaus Wolff at the 19th World Dermatology Congress in Sydney (15–20 June 1997) is highly instructive, as it relates the relative frequency of the major dermatoses to the stage in regional development.

PREVENTION TARGETS IN DERMATOLOGY	
INDUSTRIALIZED WORLD	**DEVELOPING WORLD**
◆ Skin cancer	◆ Bacterial dermatoses
◆ Occupational dermatoses	◆ Mycoses (including deep mycoses)
◆ Psoriasis	
◆ Atopic dermatitis	
◆ Skin aging and photoaging	◆ Parasitic dermatoses

AIDS
Sexually transmitted
diseases

I. DERMATOSES CAUSED BY SUNLIGHT, ULTRAVIOLET RADIATION AND X-RAYS

This chapter covers various types of skin lesions caused by sunlight, ultraviolet radiation (UVR) and X-rays. They vary greatly, as can be seen from the illustrations.

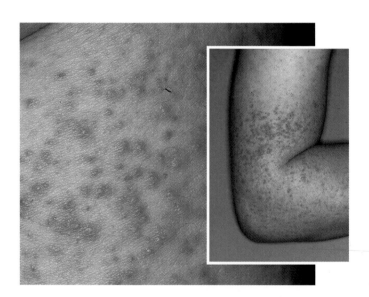

POLYMORPHIC LIGHT ERUPTION

Crops of small pruritic erythematous papules or vesicles on the extensor aspects of the upper limbs and neckline, more rarely the dorsa of the hands and feet (Photos 1 and 2).
It is most frequent in young women on their first annual exposure to bright sunlight.

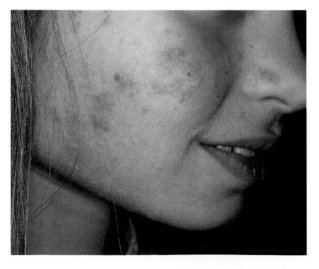

POLYMORPHIC LIGHT ERUPTION
(winter variant)

Erythematous papules on the cheeks of a small girl after her first day's exposure to mountain sunlight during a winter sports holiday.

Stratospheric ozone depletion (SOD) due to chlorofluorocarbons has long been predicted. Recent investigations demonstrate that the ozone layer shows definite thinning. Estimates suggest that ozone destruction will be enhanced for at least the next 70 years. SOD threatens to increase exposure to ultraviolet radiation in the range from 290-320 nm (UVB) reaching the surface of the earth, which is known to be a factor in a number of diseases including skin abnormalities: photoaging, photocarcinogenesis, alteration of the immune system of the skin. There is little doubt that cumulative exposure to UV-radiations is important in the aetiology of non-melanoma skin cancers. Evidence is also strong for a link with cutaneous malignant melanoma; also here it appears to be intermittent intense exposure that is most damaging.

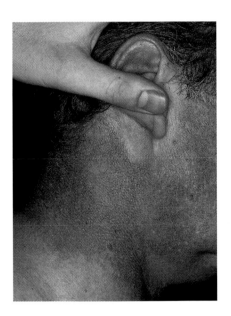

CHRONIC ACTINIC DERMATITIS

Large, variably edematous, and extremely pruritic erythematous plaque over the exposed parts of the face and neck. The retroauricular region is spared. Though often a photosensitization reaction to a drug, plant or cosmetic, it does not disappear after allergen withdrawal but persists in its own right over a prolonged period.

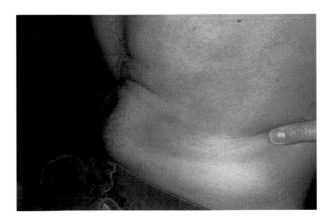

SOLAR URTICARIA

Extensive edematous erythema, with a wealing component readily apparent on digital traction. Solar urticaria is very rare, and appears minutes after exposure to sunlight. The eruption may last 3–4 hours.

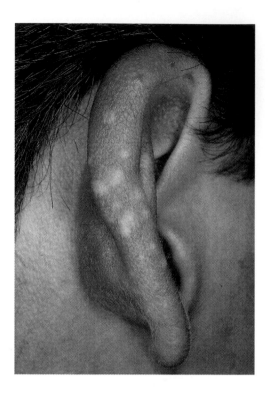

SPRING PHOTODERMATITIS OF THE EARS

A highly specific dermatosis primarily involving the ears and characterized by vesicles, preceded by pruritus, typically occurring in (mainly male) adolescents and young adults as a result of exposure to a combination of light and cold.

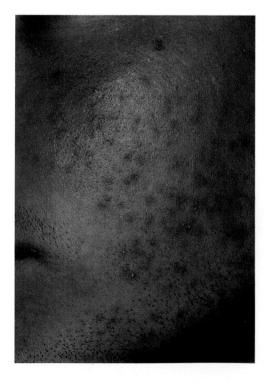

ACNE AESTIVALIS (MALLORCA ACNE)

Though sunlight generally improves acne by reducing the inflammatory component, it may in rare cases cause exacerbations.

CHRONIC (DISCOID) LUPUS ERYTHEMATOSUS

Erythematous plaques (Photo 1) covered with adherent, predominantly follicular, hyperkeratosis (Photo 2), on exposed parts, particularly the face.
Usually exacerbated by repeated exposure to sunlight, hence commoner in summer.

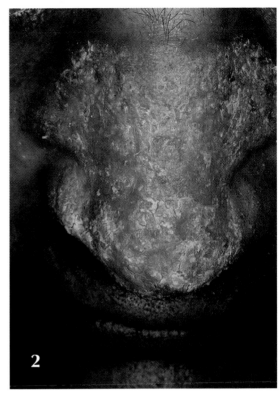

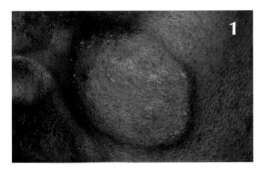

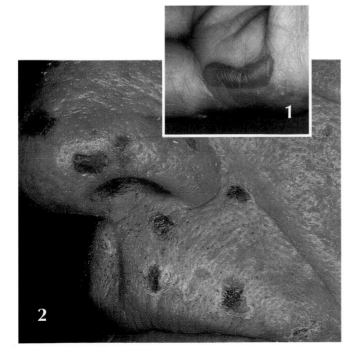

PORPHYRIA CUTANEA TARDA

The typical features are serous bullae (Photo 1) or hemorrhagic bullae and erosions (Photo 2) in reaction to sunlight on exposed parts (face and dorsa of hands, in particular). Resolution may leave scars with milia.

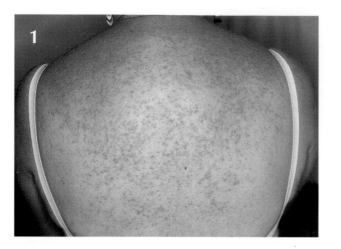

DARIER'S DISEASE

An autosomal dominant condition characterized by multiple small dry gray-brown keratotic papules which are strongly adherent (Photo 1). The papules may coalesce into extensive brownish plaques (Photo 2). The lesions are often exacerbated in summer due to the effect of sun, heat and perspiration.

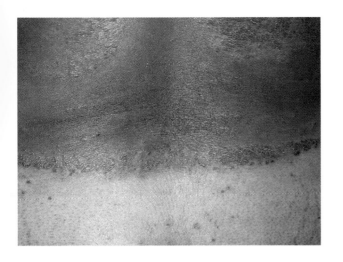

POST-PUVA EXACERBATION OF PSORIASIS

Photochemotherapy with an oral psoralen followed by long-wave UV radiation (PUVA) is a standard treatment for psoriasis but in this case has had the reverse effect, causing a shower of guttate psoriasis on the non treatment-exposed regions that can be viewed as a instance of the Köbner effect.

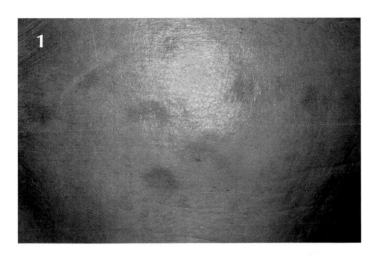

ACTINIC GRANULOMA
(O'Brien's granuloma)

Erythematous, annular and migratory lesions with giant cell dermal infiltration on the face and neck (Photo 1). The histology shows elasto-clasis, accounting for the whitish depressed scarring seen clearly in Photo 2. Sunlight appears to play a primary triggering role.

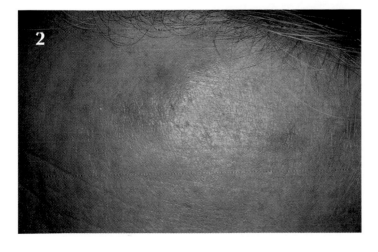

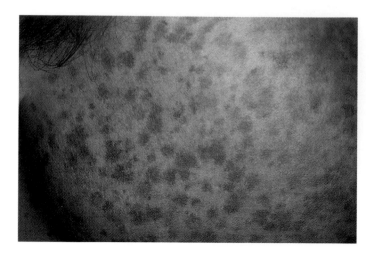

EPHELIDES (FRECKLES)

Small macules (a few mm in diameter) of pale-brown or ochre hyperpigmentation, usually appearing in childhood and thereafter permanent, but increasing in number with age and darkening on exposure to sunlight.

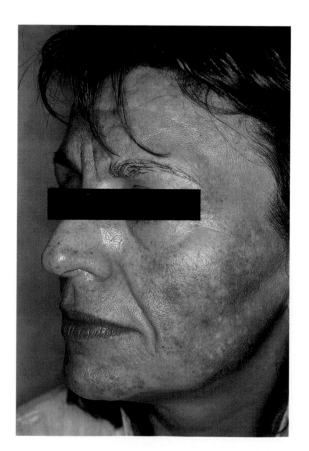

MELASMA (CHLOASMA)

Melasma is facial hyper-melanosis in women; its sites of predilection are the temples and forehead.
It is generally bilateral but never exactly symmetrical. Pregnancy and oral contraceptives are the primary determinants, and exacerbation by sunlight is well-recognized. Prevention requires the use of high factor sunscreens.

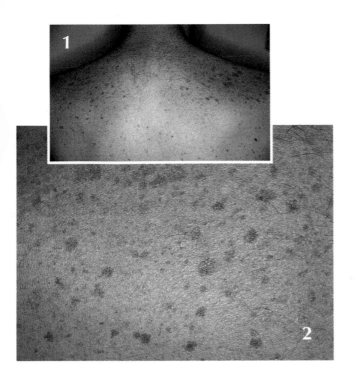

SOLAR LENTIGO (ACUTE)

Pigmented macules of varying sizes ranging from ochre to dark brown, predominantly on the shoulders and upper back (Photo 1). The mechanism is epidermal hypermelanosis (Photo 2) induced by excessive exposure to sunlight on one or more occasions.

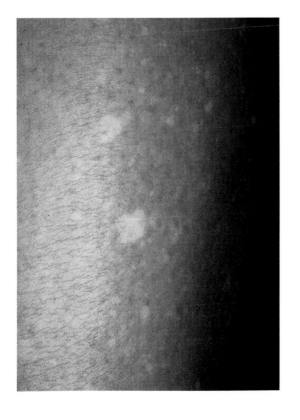

IDIOPATHIC GUTTATE HYPOMELANOSIS

Circular or oval porcelain white macules, usually a few mm in diameter, due to a decrease in epidermal melanin content after repeated exposure to UVR. Commoner in women than in men.

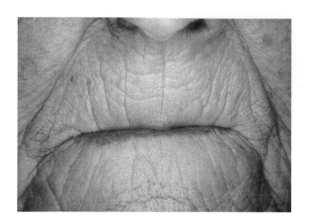

PHOTOAGING

Features include: yellowness; elastotic thickening; deep, vertical and parallel wrinkling; and retraction of the vermilion zone of the lips.

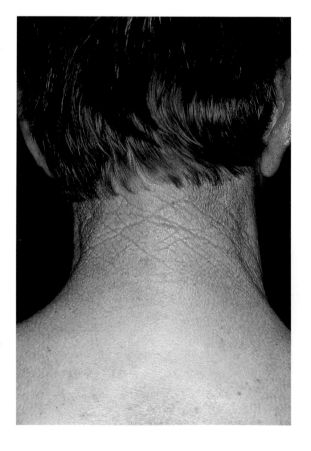

CUTIS RHOMBOIDALIS NUCHAE

A form of actinic elastosis in which deep furrows run in the thickened rhomboidal skin on the back of the neck and intersect to form yellowish diamond shapes of various sizes. It is seen mainly in subjects exposed to sun and bad weather (sailors, farmers).

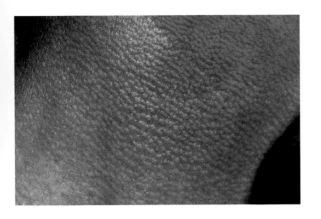

ERYTHROSIS INTERFOLLICULARIS COLLI (LEDER)

This photoaging reaction involves the anterolateral surfaces of the neck, but not the submental triangle. An extensive bright-red network of telangiectases is dotted with tiny yellowish papules (= hypertrophic sebaceous glands). It is commoner in women than in men, particularly in persons whose work or leisure has involved prolonged life-long exposure to sunlight.

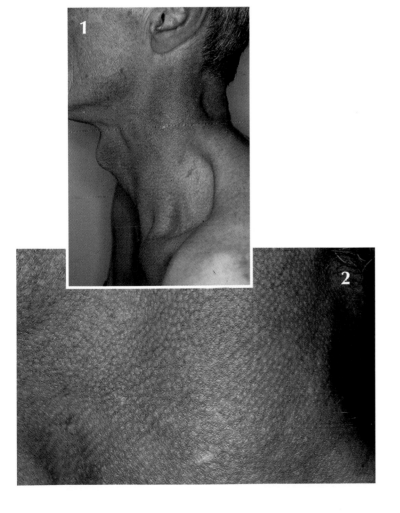

WELDERS' CHRONIC ERYTHEMA

Chronic erythema of the neck (Photo 1) in an arc welder exposed to various wavelengths of ultraviolet radiation, including UVC in some cases. Clinically, the lesions (Photo 2) resemble Leder's *erythrosis interfollicularis colli.*

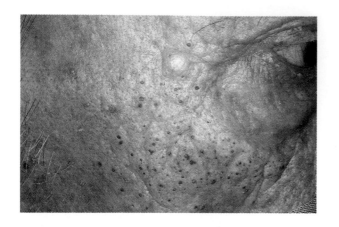

ACTINIC ELASTOSIS WITH PERIORBITAL CYSTS AND COMEDONES (FAVRE-RACOUCHOT SYNDROME)

Large prominent comedones are shown in conjunction with nodular cysts on the temporal and malar regions against a background of actinic elastosis.

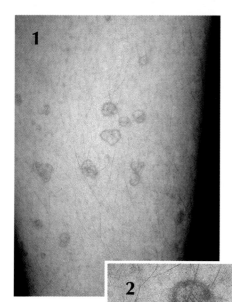

DISSEMINATED SUPERFICIAL ACTINIC POROKERATOSIS

Multiple small circular brownish lesions (Photo 1), 2–5 mm in diameter, encircled by a discretely raised keratotic ring (Photo 2) which is more palpable than visible. The lesions are found mainly on exposed areas, particularly the extensor aspects of the legs and forearms. Exacerbation occurs in summer, on exposure to sunlight, followed by regression in winter, and year-on multiplication.

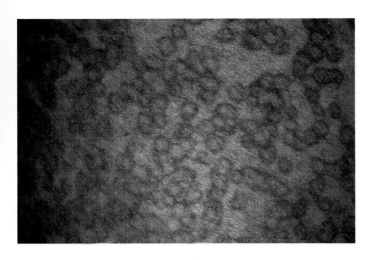

DISSEMINATED SUPERFICIAL POST-PUVA POROKERATOSIS

A variant of superficial disseminated porokeratosis developing on the entire skin surface as a rare iatrogenic complication to several sessions of PUVA therapy.

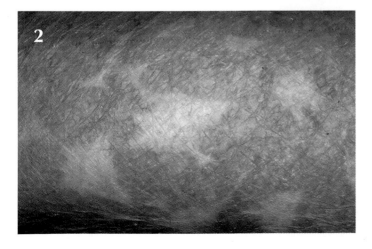

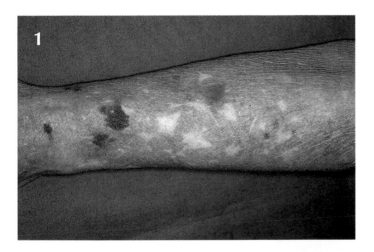

SPONTANEOUS STELLATE PSEUDOSCARRING

Milky-white pseudoscars (Photo 1) in the form of star-shaped marks (Photo 2) that stand out against the neighboring pigmented atrophic skin. They are often associated with Bateman's purpura (Photo 1). They occur in the elderly, on the extensor aspects of the forearms and dorsa of the hands. They constitute a clinical variant of skin photoaging and are exacerbated by topical and systemic steroid therapy.

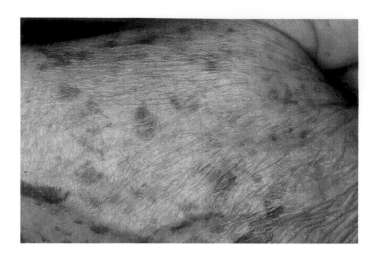

SOLAR LENTIGO (CHRONIC)

Occasionally profuse circular or oval brownish macules on the dorsa of the hands, forearms and face, due to epidermal hypermelanosis. They generally respond well to cryotherapy.

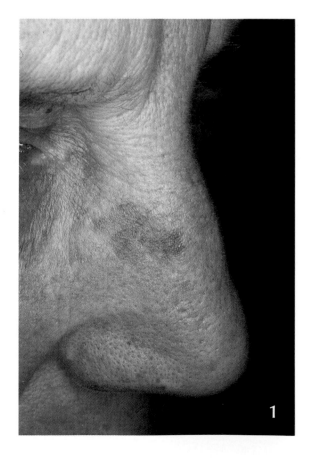

SOLAR KERATOSIS

A reaction to repeated exposure to sunlight common in those in outdoor occupations, e.g. farmers, forestry workers, builders, sailors etc. It is even commoner, and often multiple, in those who have lived in the tropics. Clinical presentations vary: some lesions are flat, slightly keratotic, erythematous plaques with well-defined margins (Photo 1).

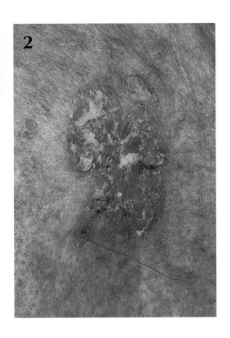

Bowenoid solar keratosis is a red-brown variant with sharp but irregular margins.
The lesions are slightly raised, with thin adherent scales.
The surrounding skin is scattered with telangiectatic capillaries – another clinical feature of photoaging (Photo 2).

Horn induration, a localized accumulation of keratin usually on the face or ears, is another classical variant (Photo 3).

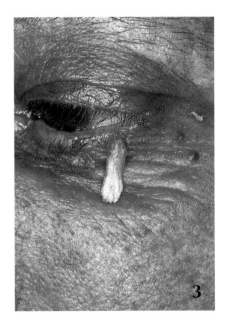

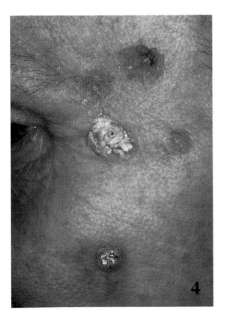

Facial photoaging sometimes presents as a combination of actinic and seborrheic keratosis (Photo 4).

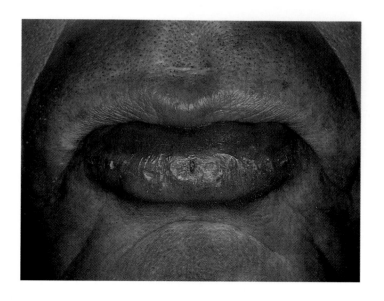

ACTINIC CHEILITIS

An erythematous crusting band extending along the length of the lower lip. It constitutes actinic keratosis of the lip and can thus degenerate into invasive squamous carcinoma.
The lower lip is more commonly involved due to its greater exposure to sunlight.

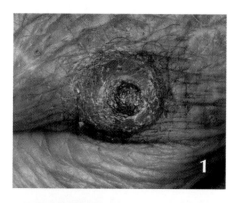

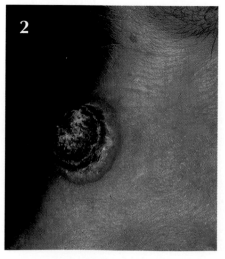

KERATO-ACANTHOMA

A firm sharply marginated nodule containing a central horny plug found mainly on skin regions chronically exposed to sunlight.
It grows rapidly to maximal size in a few weeks (Photo 1). Regression is normally spontaneous (Photo 2) and complete after a few months. Human papilloma-virus (HPV) and other viruses are possible cofactors in the pathogenesis.

NODULAR BASAL CELL CARCINOMA

Globular smooth-surfaced tumor covered with fine telangiectases. Facial photoaging is a major contributory factor.

BASAL CELL CARCINOMA (RODENT ULCER)

This tumor is characterized by marked downward "rodent" spread and a persistent translucent pearly margin.

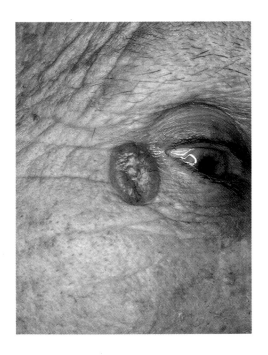

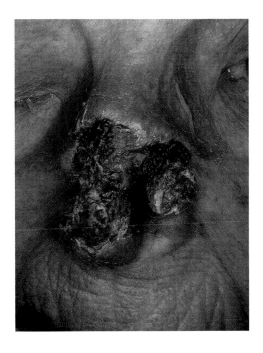

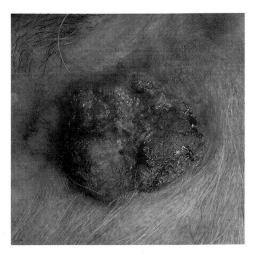

SQUAMOUS CELL CARCINOMA

A deeply indurated, ulcerating and bleeding tumor mass on the temple. The entire lesion base is heavily infiltrated.

CUTANEOUS MELANOMA AND THE ENVIRONMENT

Exposure to sunlight is closely associated with the development of melanoma, and is the cause of two thirds of cases. Mode of exposure is also important: intermittent exposure, e.g. on holiday, at weekends or during leisure pursuits, is more closely associated with melanoma than regular exposure as in those who work outdoors. However, these generalizations are not mutually exclusive.

UVA and UVB are primarily responsible: sunbeds mainly generate UVA and thus may be a risk factor. The illustrations show only a few clinical aspects of melanoma.

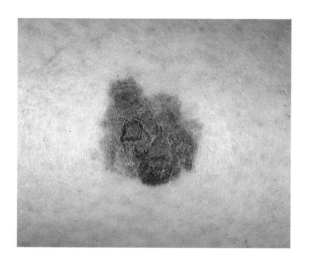

SUPERFICIAL SPREADING MELANOMA

Melanotic brown to black lesion with polycyclic borders. This slightly raised tumor is spreading laterally but has entered its vertically downward invasive phase, producing a small central pink nodule.

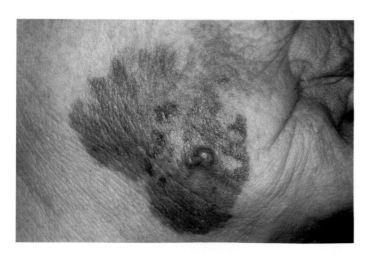

LENTIGO MALIGNA MELANOMA (PREMALIGNANT MELANOSIS OF DUBREUILH)

A large flat pigmented polychromic macule, ranging from light beige to dark brown, with irregular margins. A small, red, easily bleeding nodule indicates downward spread.

MELANOMA: DERMATOSCOPY (EPILUMINESCENCE)

Three diagnostic dermatoscopic signs in an early Clark II melanoma (Breslow thickness index: 0.25 mm):

a) blue-white veil;

b) peripheral brown dots;

c) reversed pigment network.

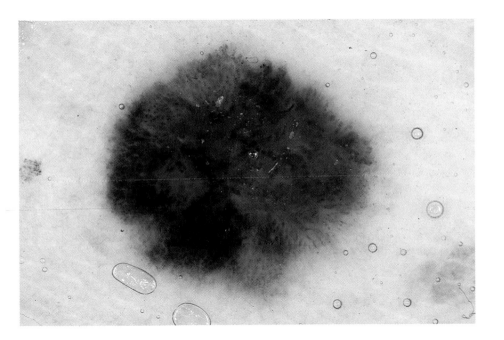

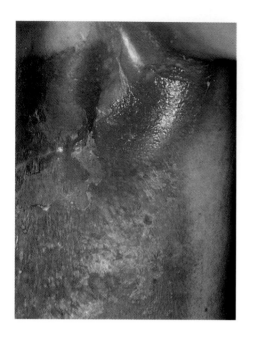

ACUTE RADIODERMATITIS

Extensive erythematous exudative plaque typical of acute radiodermatitis, following a dose of 10–20 Gy.

POST-THERAPEUTIC RADIODERMATITIS

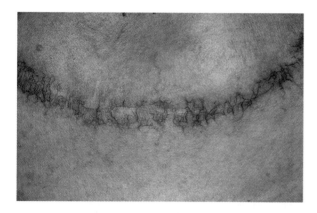

Thyroidectomy and radiotherapy for thyroid cancer: active development of a fine network of telangiectases associated with atrophy and depigmentation as the only signs of chronic minimal radiodermatitis.

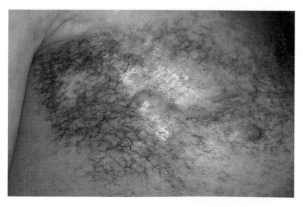

Massive irradiation for breast cancer: extensive chronic radiodermatitis comprising large areas of atrophy, depigmentation, and an extensive network of telangiectases.

OCCUPATIONAL RADIODERMATITIS

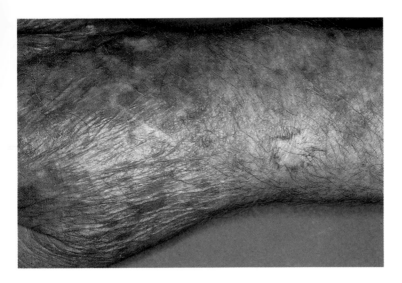

Chronic radiodermatitis on the dorsum of the hand in a radiologist. The features include cicatricial atrophy, telangiectasia and abnormal pigmentation (areas of hypermelanosis and depigmentation).

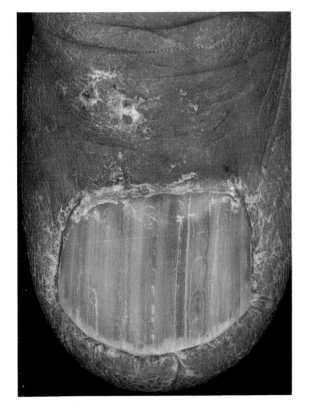

Chronic radiodermatitis on a dentist's finger. Skin atrophy on the tip of the phalanx with small precancerous keratoses. The longitudinal striae and altered lunula are evidence of nail involvement.

Modern use of proper protection has made these conditions exceptional.

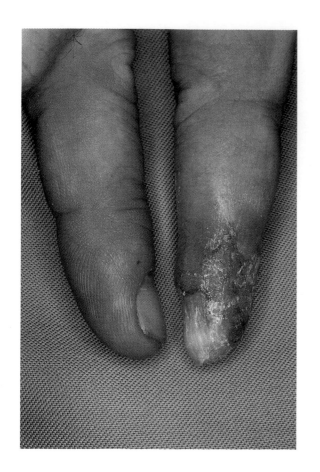

BOWEN'S DISEASE (INTRA-EPIDERMAL CARCINOMA)

Erosive, scaly or crusty erythematous plaque with slightly raised edges invading the entire fingertip following radiodermatitis in a radiologist. Untreated Bowen's disease progresses gradually to invasive carcinoma.

II. DERMATOSES CAUSED BY ENVIRONMENTAL HYGROMETRY AND TEMPERATURE CONDITIONS

ERYTHEMA AB IGNE

The initial features are erythema and reticular telangiectasia which gradually progress to an irreversible ochre or brown pigmentation. The cause is prolonged exposure of the body part to a strong heat source. The evidence is that infrared radiation is primarily responsible, its effects being combined with that of the specific heat factor.

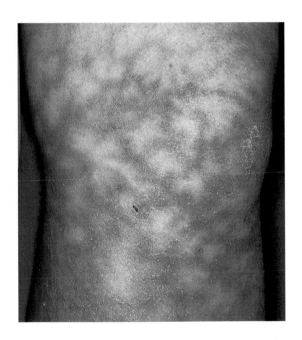

Lesions at the erythema-telangiectasia stage on the medial aspects of the lower limbs after repeated exposure to an outdoor heater at a winter market.

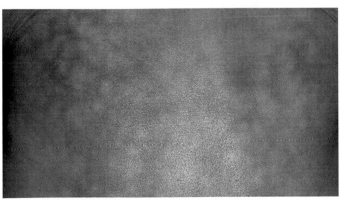

Advanced pigmented lesions in an elderly person after repeated exposure of the back to an electric radiator.

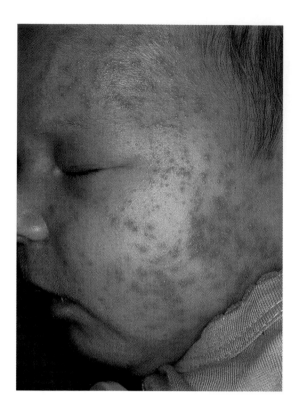

NEONATAL MILIARIA RUBRA (PRICKLY HEAT)

Very frequently observed in infants.
Crops of erythematous vesicles on an infant's cheeks and forehead in response to an overheated environment.

MILIARIA CRYSTALLINA

Crops of small, clear, non pruritic vesicles 1–2 mm in diameter appear mainly on the trunk, due to blockade of the intra-epidermal portion of the sweat ducts, typically in humid heat, e.g. the tropics. Excessively tight-fitting working garments are responsible for the occupational variant.

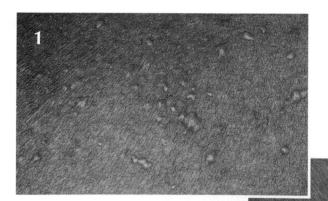

Photo 1. Miliaria crystallina after a day's exposure in a tropical resort.

Photo 2. Miliaria crystallina on a background of diffuse erythema during a trip to Africa.

HYPERHIDROSIS

Hyperhidrosis can be generalized or localized to a well-defined area of skin, e.g. axilla, palm, and sole. Whichever the area involved, the condition is a major handicap in everyday life, during work, sport, or strenuous leisure pursuits. Emotional stress is a particular determinant of palmar hyperhidrosis.

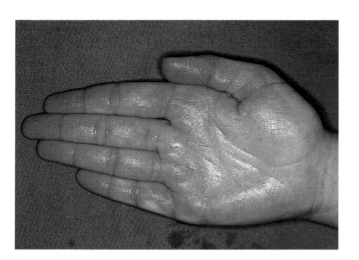

PALMAR HYPERHIDROSIS

The hands run with sweat, and there is associated mild acrocyanosis (Photo 1). This is an extreme case, most instances of hyperhidrosis simply involving sweatiness of the hands.

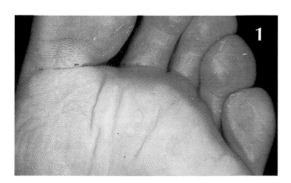

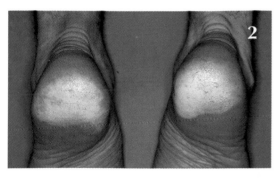

PLANTAR HYPERHIDROSIS

The distinctive feature is maceration: the sodden cyanotic skin can be fissured to varying depths, making walking painful. It is most marked at pressure points and usually symmetrical. It often causes bromhidrosis (malodorous perspiration) due to microbial proliferation, and may be associated with pitted keratolysis.

Photo 1.
Forefoot hyperhidrosis with deep furrows causing pain on walking.

Photo 2.
Selective hyperhidrosis of the heels, perhaps due to an eccrine hamartoma in an area of high sweat gland density.

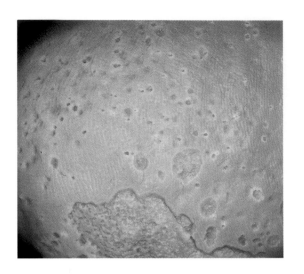

PITTED KERATOLYSIS

Shallow circular erosions of the corneal layer with a punched-out appearance, mainly in plantar pressure-bearing areas, with associated loss of the skin lines, usually but not always in the presence of hyperhidrosis. The condition is due to the presence of filamentous Gram-positive organisms (*Streptomyces spp.* and *Corynebacterium spp.*) found in the erosion "wells".

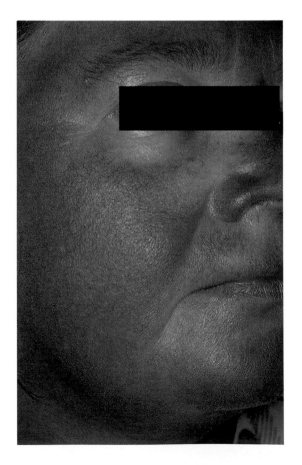

ROSACEA AND OCCUPATIONAL ENVIRONMENT

Rosacea is defined as erythema and telangiectasia of the nose, cheeks and chin. The periocular region is spared. Vasomotor flushes occur under a variety of circumstances: stress, environmental temperature change (especially from cold to hot), ingestion of alcohol or hot food and drink. Claims, particularly in Sweden, that the condition is exacerbated by exposure to VDUs have no scientific basis.

EXERTIONAL URTICARIA

Exertion may trigger generalized urticaria in some people. It is a variant of physical urticaria probably resulting from several factors, including heat and perspiration.

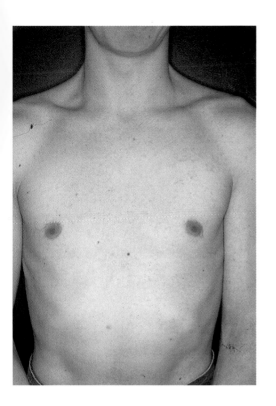

No urticaria
before exercise.

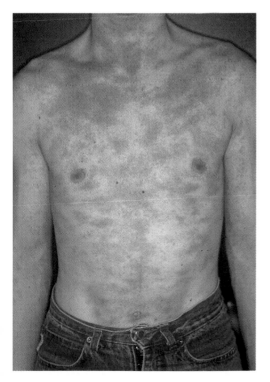

Florid urticaria
after running.

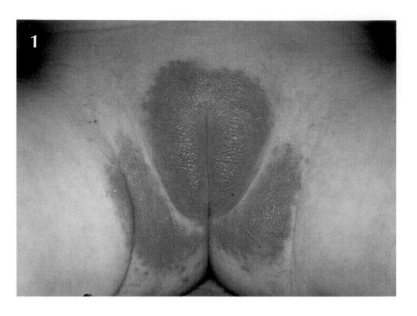

DIAPER DERMATITIS

An irritant glazed and confluent W-shaped erythema of the convex surfaces of the anogenital region of infants.

The margins may be sharp (Photo 1) or made up of isolated small papules and vesicles (Photo 2). The condition is due to prolonged confined contact with urine and feces combined with chafing.

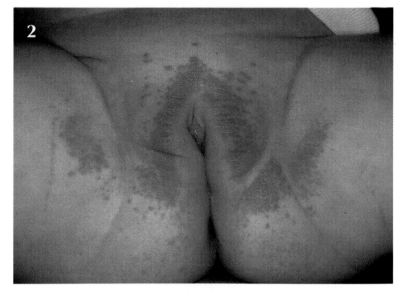

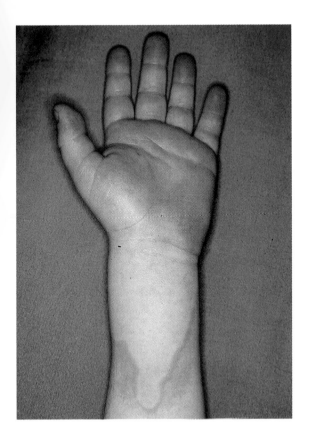

COLD URTICARIA

An extensive plaque of urticaria (Photos 1 and 2) in response to cold challenge (5 min hand immersion in water at 4 °C).

This is a case of authentic cold urticaria; aquagenic urticaria was excluded by hand immersion in water at room temperature.

Cold urticaria can be a considerable occupational handicap for those working in a cold environment (e.g. cold storage plants) or who put their hands into cold water. In the latter case, the hands become violently pruritic and edematous, with limited flexion and extension.

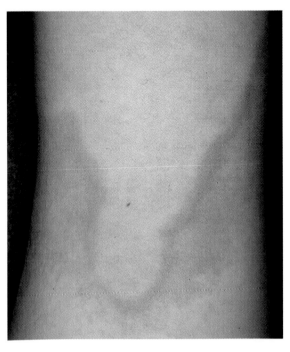

COLD PANNICULITIS

Subcutaneous purplish and painful plaques due to extensive inflammatory induration of hypodermal fat tissue. It occurs in winter, during work or sport. It is commoner in women and is seen mainly on the thighs, knees and proximal third of the leg.

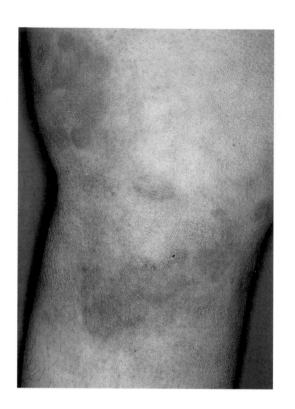

Occupational panniculitis of the medial aspect of the thighs and legs in a female market gardener.

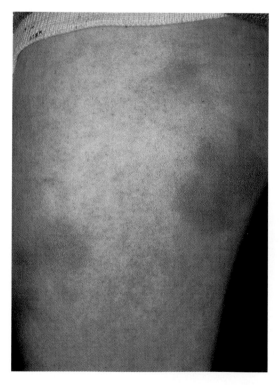

Panniculitis of the lateral aspect of the thigh in a horsewoman.

ACROCYANOSIS

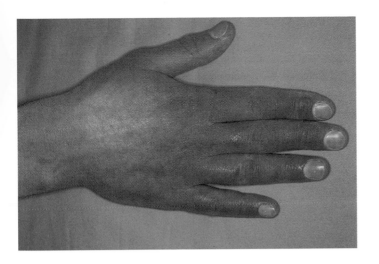

Permanent and painless purplish-blue discoloration of the extremities, mainly in girls. The occupational environment may contribute, particularly when the hands are often exposed to dry or damp cold.

RAYNAUD'S SYNDROME

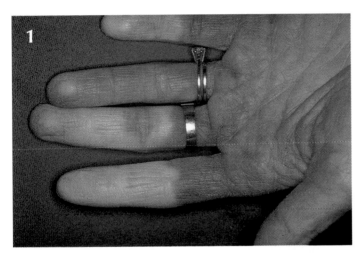

The hands are symmetrically affected, and sometimes the feet. Cold precipitates sudden pallor, with one or more fingers becoming cold, mottled and numb; the upper limit of the vasospasm is clear, on the first phalanges.

After a few minutes, pallor is followed by cyanosis and pain.

Raynaud's syndrome may be isolated (Photo 1) or part of systemic sclerosis (scleroderma) (Photo 2) in which case it is associated with necrotic ulceration.

It is the major symptom of occupational vibration syndrome.

CHILBLAINS (PERNIOSIS)

Chilblains are localized erythematous or erythrocyanotic lesions of the extremities which may be covered in clear or hemorrhagic bullae, or ulceration and crusts. Purple and painful in the cold, they turn bright red and become pruritic on entry into the warm. They occur mainly in cold humid climates in subjects exposed to cold in their working lives. They typically recur every winter, with remission only in summer.

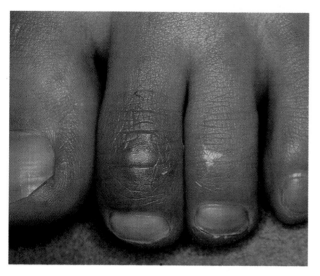

Purplish erythematous infiltrated lesions of the toes.

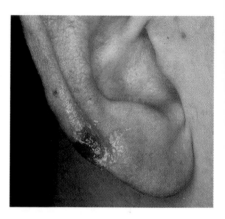

Crusty ulceration on the free border of the ear.

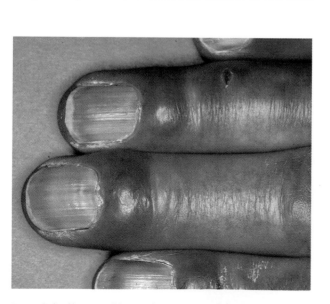

Pseudobullous infiltrated periungual lesions.

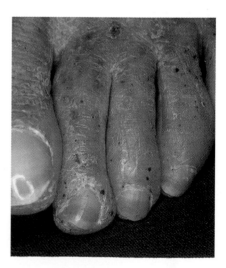

Crusty erythrocyanotic lesions due to cryoglobulinemia (cold agglutinins).

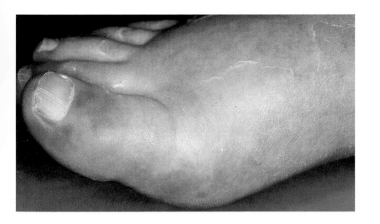

FROSTBITE

Extensive cyanotic and painful erythematous area on the forefoot after an expedition at altitude during a winter sports holiday. The regression phase has commenced, as shown by the line of desquamation on the dorsum of the foot.

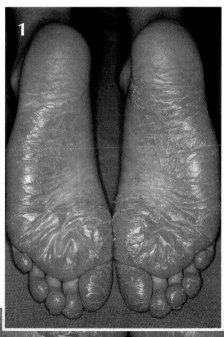

JUVENILE PLANTAR DERMATOSIS

This childhood condition arises in plantar surface of the forefoot (Photo 1); it is always bilateral and usually symmetrical. It is characterized by the triad of erythema, hyperkeratosis and fissures. The skin often becomes glazed and mildly macerated (Photo 2). Winter exacerbation is typical.

The etiopathogenesis is unknown, but is probably multifactorial (a combination of genetic and environmental factors).

The corneal layer is probably weakened and dehydrated by sudden changes in temperature and humidity: during the day, children wear occlusive footwear (high-ankle trainers), promoting maceration, while at night they are exposed to a warm dry (centrally heated) environment.

ECZEMA CRAQUELÉ (ASTEATOTIC ECZEMA)

Generally found on an excessively dry skin, in particular in the elderly during cold dry winters, mainly on the legs and thighs, and more rarely the trunk.
The illustrations show different phases:

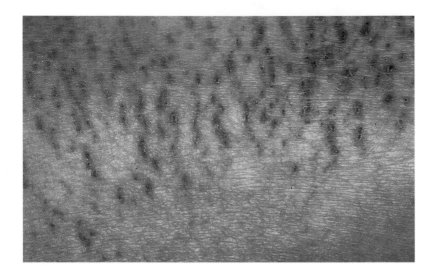

Simple erythema craquelé, with roughly parallel cracks of varying depth.

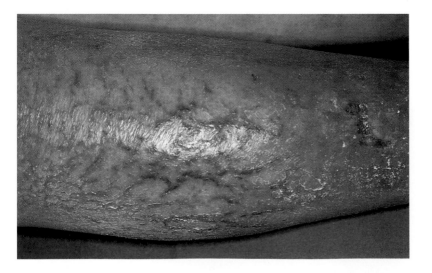

The cracks are deeper and run in all directions, in a crazy-paving pattern. Some are prone to bleed.

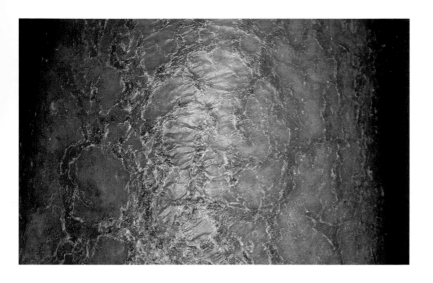

Cracks on a diffuse erythematosquamous background: this is the appearance that gave rise to the term eczema craquelé.

Erythema craquelé is a well-recognized complication of various ichthyotic (fish scale-like) conditions and is explained by the specific features of the corneal layer in these conditions.

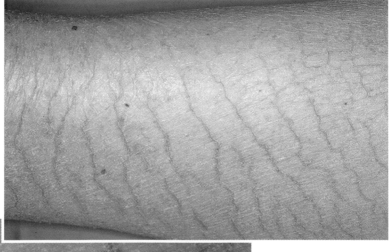

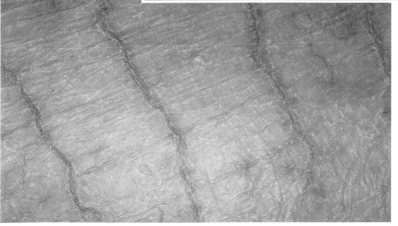

III. DERMATOSES CAUSED BY MECHANICAL FACTORS AND/OR TRAUMA

ACANTHOMA FISSURATUM

A reactive skin nodule, primarily of the epidermis (hence the name acanthoma), following repeated friction from a hard object.

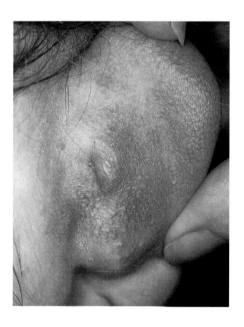

SPECTACLE FRAME ACANTHOMA FISSURATUM

Ear: a well-circumscribed pinkish retroauricular nodule grooved along one border, occurring weeks or months after a change of spectacle frame.

Nose: a bright red nodule with a central circular ulcer depression due to spectacle frame friction, especially if the frame is heavy. The lesion has become much rarer with light modern frames.

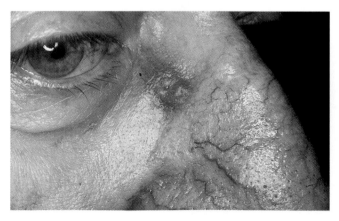

ENDOBUCCAL ACANTHOMA FISSURATUM

Elongated verrucous lesion which is whitish from maceration, showing a deep and painful slit along its length. The cause was repeated friction from a metal orthodontic device.

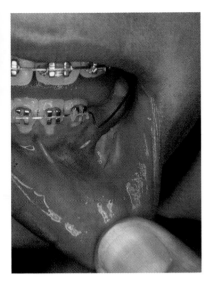

CHONDRODERMATITIS NODULARIS ANTHELICIS

A degenerative lesion of the dermis and underlying cartilage favouring the mid part of the antihelix of the ear. Exquisitely tender, it begins as a small papulonodule which is necrotic at its center, under an adherent crust (Photo 1). It gradually increases in size to an oblong nodule with central ulcerated depression (Photo 2).
The main cause appears to be friction, particularly from hats fitting tightly around the ears. Other factors – heat, radiation, and advancing age – may play only a negligible role in this variant of painful nodule of the ear (in contrast to their probably major contribution to *chondrodermatitis nodularis helicis*).

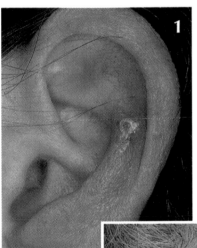

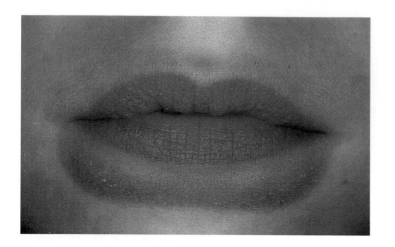

LICK ECZEMA

A mechanical pericheilitis caused by persistent licking, a habit tic common in children : the brownish sharply marginated band is slightly squamous around the lips and particularly florid on the chin.

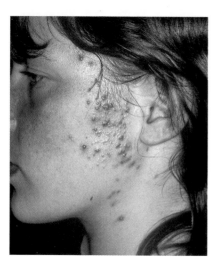

MECHANICAL ACNE

It is not unusual for the papulopustular lesions in acne to be more marked at pressure and friction points. In this case – a girl moped rider – the lesions are concentrated in a preauricular rectangle with a vertical main axis, i.e. the area occluded by her crash helmet.

In sports medicine, mechanical acne is seen on the neck and shoulders in American football players, hockey players, golfers and female aerobics enthusiasts.

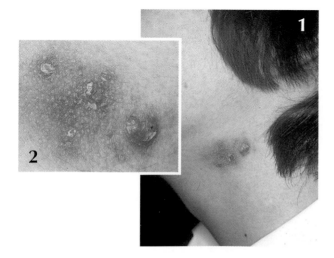

FIDDLER'S NECK

Long plaque of lichenification on the left side of the face at the point where the chin rest presses against the skin over the angle of the jaw (Photo 1). Papulopustular lesions, which are occasionally nodulocystic and similar to those in mechanical acne, may develop on the plaque (Photo 2).

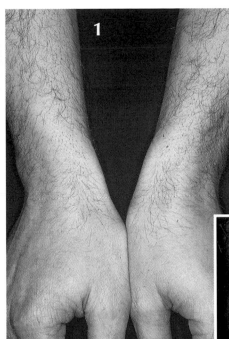

FRICTION HYPOTRICHOSIS

Constant limb skin friction in men, whether by clothing or repeated movement at work or in sport, causes reversible wear-and-tear hypotrichosis. Photo 1 is a highly characteristic example on the distal extensor aspects of the forearms in a badminton player: the distribution is entirely symmetrical. A close-up shows hypotrichosis (Photo 2).

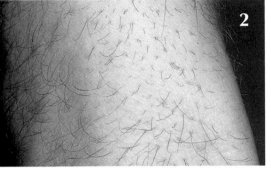

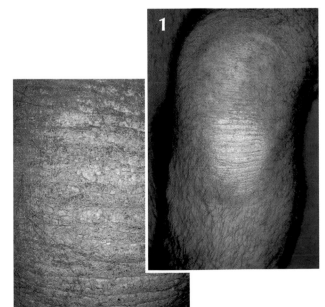

FRICTION LICHENIFICATION AND HYPERKERATOSIS OF THE KNEES

Reactive thickening of the knee skin into grayish, pink or more strongly pigmented plaques of variable size with well-defined borders (Photo 1).
The areas of keratotic thickening are sometimes arranged in parallel striae (Photo 2). The occupations typically affected are the building trades, in particular tiling and roofing.

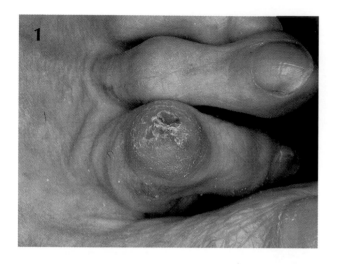

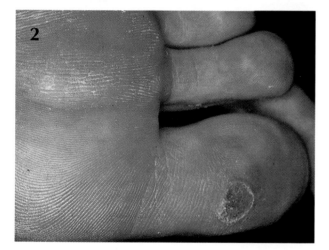

ORTHOPEDIC CALLOSITIES

These are found only on the feet and are extremely common. They fall into three distinct groups :

corns (Photo 1) are localized callosities shaped like an upside-down cone with the hyperkeratotic spike resting on a small area of bone, subject to permanent friction. They are most usual on the dorsal surface of the interphalangeal joints and often exquisitely painful.

plantar callosities (Photo 2) occur on the plantar or lateral aspect of the feet as plaques of yellowish hyperkeratosis of varying thickness, which are painful on walking. They are caused by repeated friction, as bone and joint deformities gradually alter the pressure points. The photograph illustrates the clinical characteristics differentiating a callosity on the plantar vault (the skin lines are retained) and a viral wart on the plantar aspect of the big toe (loss of the skin lines and presence of black dots).

heel callosities (Photo 3) are very common, particularly in the elderly. They consist of hyperkeratotic and variably fissured plaques.

In all three cases, the friction is due to shoes which fail to espouse the architecture of the foot.

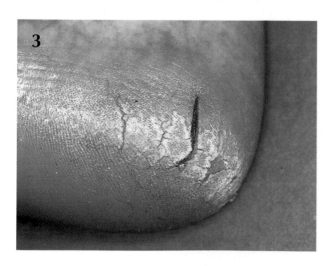

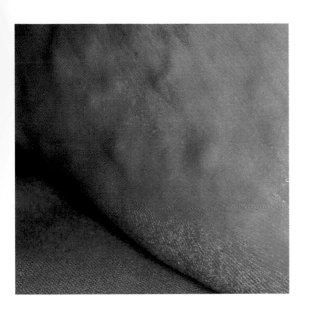

PIEZOGENIC PEDAL PAPULES

Herniation of subcutaneous fat into the dermis on the lateral aspect of the heel. The prevalence may be as high as 10–20 % of the population, with women and children being most affected. The papules are skin-coloured and only visible on standing. They are generally asymptomatic. The term "painful piezogenic pedal papules" is used only for lesions causing marked discomfort and shooting pains in competitive athletes.

EPIDERMOLYSIS BULLOSA: EXACERBATION BY ENVIRONMENTAL FACTORS

Congenital epidermolysis bullosa may be simple (non dystrophic) or dystrophic.
The illustrations show simple generalized epidermolysis bullosa; bullous lesions of the knees (Photo 1) in a child, resolving without scars except for some small inclusion cysts of mat white keratin which disappear after a few weeks.
Photo 2: two tense bullae on the palm of the hand and fingers. The bullae are caused by microtrauma or repeated friction, in particular at work, sport or leisure activity, in a hot and humid environment.

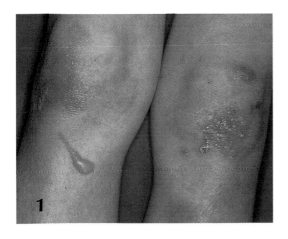

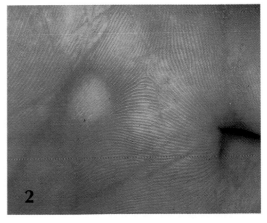

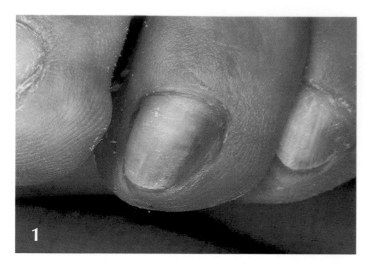

FRICTION MELANONYCHIA

A new entity described by Baran in 1987 and caused by repeated microtrauma from ill-fitting shoes.
The distinctive feature is a longitudinal brown band, usually from the lateral part of the big toenail (Photo 1). It may affect several toes and is much darker in Blacks or mixed race subjects (Photo 2). It is important to recognize: the differential diagnoses are physiological longitudinal melanonychia in Blacks (and Japanese) and, above all, the longitudinal melanonychia symptomatic of a matrix naevus or melanoma.

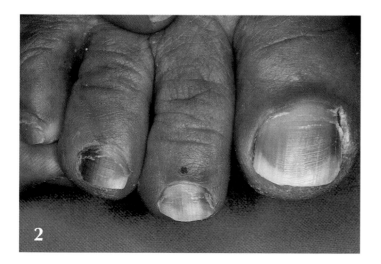

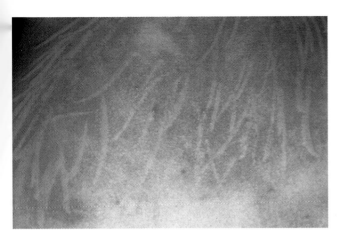

DERMOGRAPHISM

A line of edematous erythema in response to a frictional stimulus of the skin, in excess of the weal-and-flare seen in normal subjects. The photograph shows dermographism following frenzied scratching with the fingernails. It usually occurs 5–10 minutes after the frictional stimulus, though in exceptional cases it occurs later (delayed dermographism) and can be demonstrated during clinical examination by firm stroking of the skin with a blunt-pointed instrument. It may be asymptomatic or pruritic. A typical complaint by patients is intense pruritus after a bath or shower.

PRESSURE URTICARIA

Mechanical pressure urticaria is a not unexceptional variant of physical urticaria. The lesions are confined to the area subject to pressure, generally beginning 4–8 hours later. They are pruritic and sometimes painful. The case shown – a long erythematous edematous plaque on the scapular region, with some small isolated peripheral urticarial papules – was caused by a shoulder bag.
In work or sport, the lesions typically occur on the palms of the hands, the soles of the feet during walking or on the buttocks after prolonged sitting.

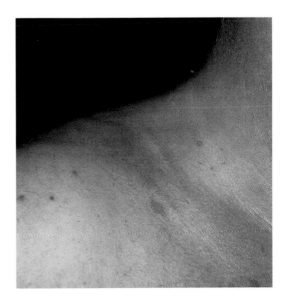

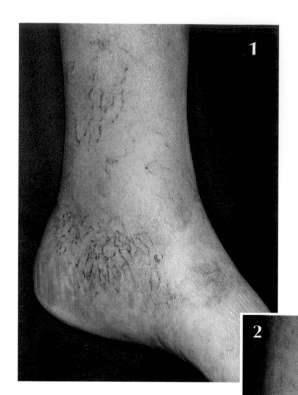

VARICES AND OCCUPATIONAL ACTIVITY

Superficial varicosities in the medial malleolar region and lower leg (Photo 1). The hypodermic varicosities follow a branching pattern (Photo 2).
The major problems are caused by more substantial varices (Photo 3).
The ergonomic data show exacerbation by occupational factors, in particular constant standing or sitting, without moving.

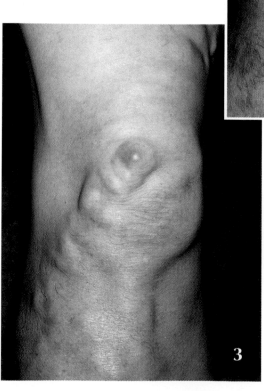

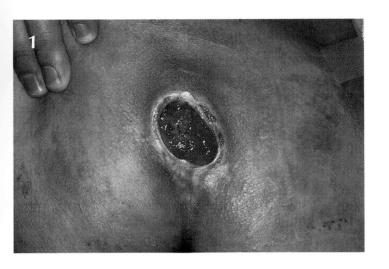

DECUBITUS ULCER

A deep, painless chronic ulcer typically at a pressure point over bone, occurring in immobilized subjects (e.g. elderly bedridden patients, younger paraplegics etc). The edge shows no tendency to spontaneous resolution or deterioration while the ulcer base displays red granulation (Photo 1). Close-up shows the characteristic open "shirt-button" appearance of the edge (Photo 2).

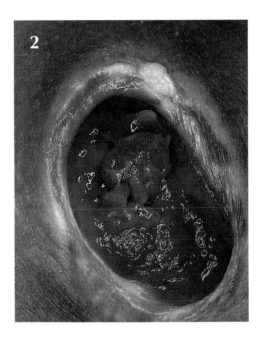

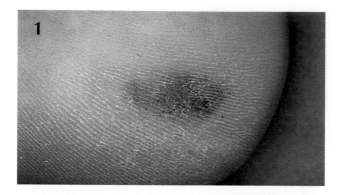

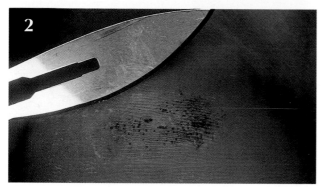

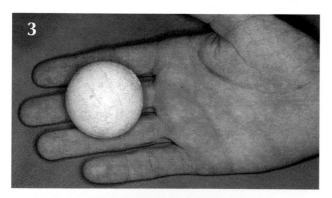

BLACK HEEL

The classic descriptions of this variant of intracorneal hematoma are from sports medicine: a confluent spangle of blackish dots due to minute hemorrhages in the papillary dermis (following capillary rupture) during exertion. Heme pigment is eliminated transepidermally; microscopy shows amorphous collections of brownish material within the stratum corneum. The most common site is the posterior or postero-lateral aspect of the heel, just above the hyperkeratotic edge of the foot, uni- or bilaterally (Photo 1). The black dots are best visualized by paring the superficial corneal layer with a scalpel (Photo 2). Sports which require sudden acceleration (basket-ball, athletics, tennis, volley ball) may have a contributory role. An identical lesion (black palm) may develop on the palm in weightlifters, golfers, tennis players or, as in the case illustrated, players of balle pelote, a popular sport in Belgium (Photo 3). In this case, the black dots are concentrated in the pit of a natural skin crease which is uniformly brownish and the focus of the microtrauma involved in catching and returning the ball (Photo 4).

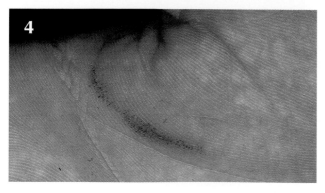

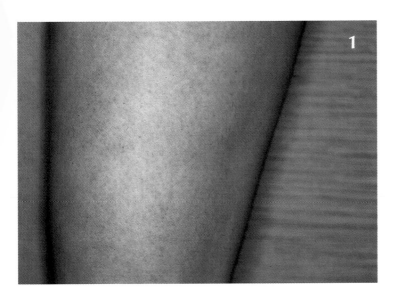

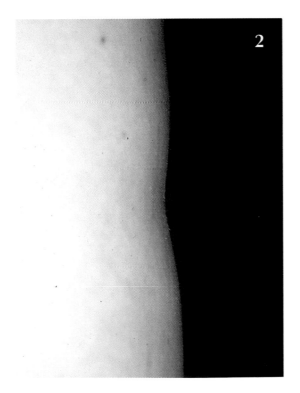

LIPOATROPHIA SEMICIRCULARIS

A band-like circular depression on the anterolateral aspects of the thighs (Photo 1), particularly in young adult women. It is best viewed in slanting natural light (Photo 2). The probable cause is the microtrauma of repeated contact with hard objects, e.g. table and desk edges, causing partial destruction of adipocyte tissue.
The microanatomy of adipocyte tissue distribution in young women may be a further contributory factor.

Psoriasis along surgical scars.

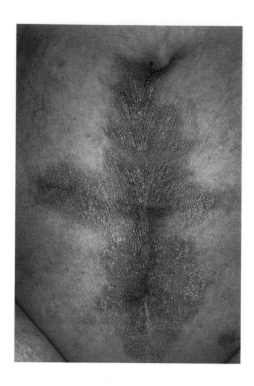

PSORIASIS AND THE KÖBNER (ISOMORPHIC) EFFECT

The Köbner (isomorphic) effect describes the induction of skin disease by physical or non specific trauma at a previously disease-free site.
It is typically observed in some subjects with psoriasis. The trauma-lesion interval is 2–3 weeks.
The term "trauma" covers wounds, burns, mechanical stimulation, and irritation by chemical agents or UVR.

Linear psoriasis in a gardener with florid psoriasis after being scratched by a prickly bush during clearing work.

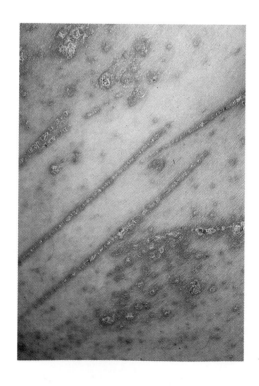

LICHEN PLANUS AND THE KÖBNER EFFECT

The Köbner effect is also seen in some subjects with active lichen planus.

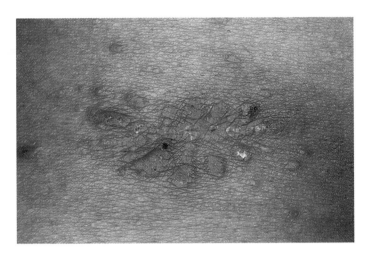

Lichen planus on a naevus excision scar. The firm purplish papules shine in slanting light and show the whitish (Wickham's) striae caused by keratotic thickening.

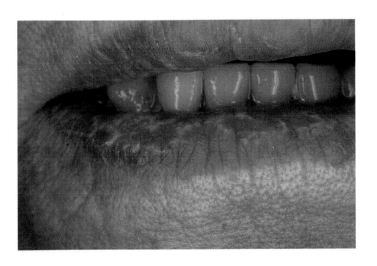

Typical lichen planus of the lower lip with a distinctive reticular appearance due to a network of white Wickham's striae.
The condition can be exacerbated by persistent gnawing and licking.

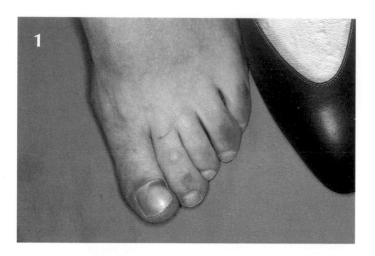

MICROTRAUMATIC ONYCHOLYSIS OF THE BIG TOENAIL

A combination of two factors is responsible : orthopedic abnormalities of the feet and ill-fitting shoes (Photo 1). Shedding progresses proximally along a posteriorly convex line resulting in a semi-lunar appearance (Photo 2). In the case shown, the lesion is surrounded by a brownish stain that is probably due to microhemorrhage (hemosiderotic pseudome-lanonychia).

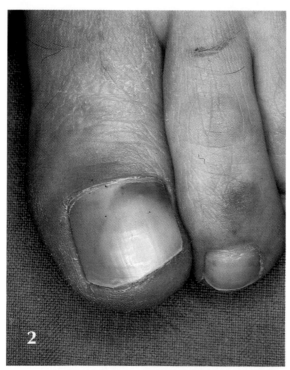

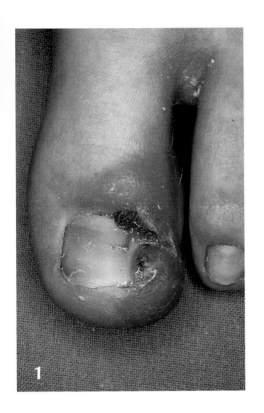

1

INGROWING TOENAIL

Ingrowing great toe nail involving an entire lateral edge of the plate and surrounded by extensive infected granulation tissue (Photo 1). Ill-fitting shoes have accelerated the process in a predisposed subject. At this stage in its course, the lesion requires radical cure: resection of the nail spicules at the edge of the nail plate and curetage of the granulation tissue as a first stage, followed by permanent selective destruction of the homologous lateral matrix in the second stage.

Photo 2: incipient ingrowing nail, which can be corrected by supportive measures enabling the nail to grow until its edges clear the end of the toe.

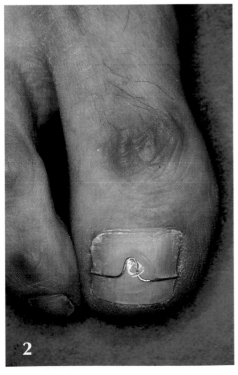

2

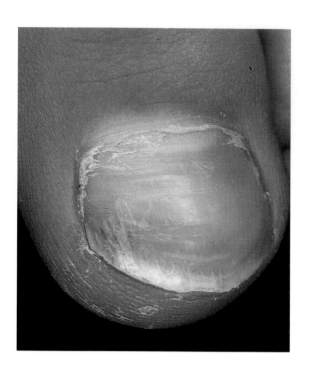

SUBUNGUAL FILIFORM (OR FLAME-SHAPED) HEMATOMA

Repeated microtrauma are responsible for these fine blackish linear stripes 2–3 mm long running along the main axis of the nails of both fingers and toes. The condition occurs in healthy subjects but also in many conditions sharing an increased susceptibility of the capillary bed to microtrauma.

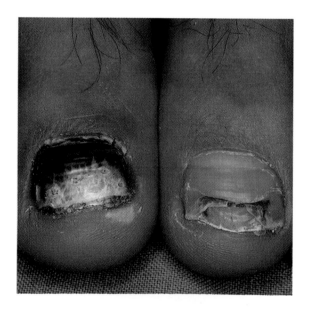

JOGGER'S TOE

Repeated microtrauma cause toe nail lesions, in particular of the great toe. Several variants are shown in this photograph of an extreme case: distal onycholysis with fragmentation of the nail plate, hyperkeratosis of the nail bed, extensive hematoma. The nail is often shed. Most cases are milder. The sports usually responsible are jogging, tennis, football, rugby, basketball, volleyball, hockey, mountain climbing and skiing.

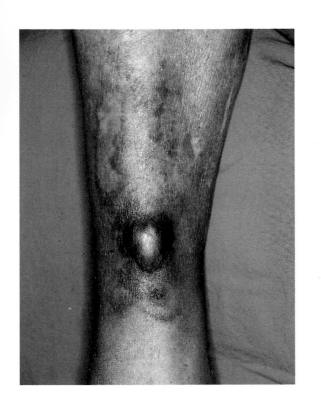

TRAUMATIC HEMATOMA OF THE LEG

After a direct blow, there is a painful variably sized collection of blood which dissects skin tissue and muscle masses. A drainage incision is often necessary. A variant is traumatic hematoma of the shoulder which in this site has to be differentiated from spontaneous hematoma.

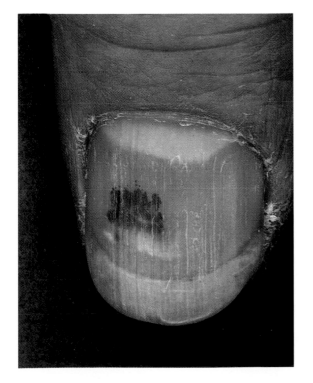

SUBUNGUAL HEMATOMA

An irregularly marginated, blackish or deep purple stain under the nail plate, with dot microhemorrhages around the edges. The cause is trauma and most lesions migrate over a few months to the distal extremity of the nail. In rarer cases, no migration takes place: the fixed hematoma differs from a naevus or other nail pigmentation in its deep purple color, irregular outline, and absence of coloration in the nail keratin itself.

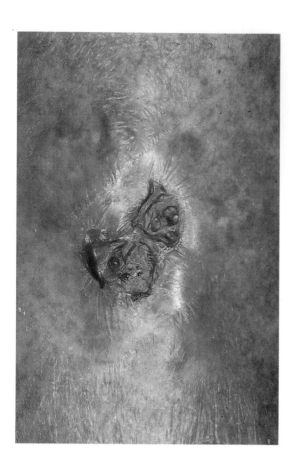

POSTTRAUMATIC VENOUS ULCER

There are fissures in the ulcer edges and multiple phleboliths (small calcium concretions found in the walls of varicose veins) in the ulcer base.

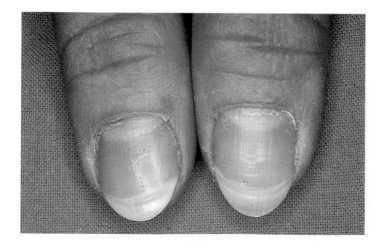

MANICURE ONYCHOLYSIS

Onycholysis due to over-enthusiastic manicure is very common in women. It is characterized by opaque detachment of the nail, with a proximal border that is linear in the present case, but wavy in others.

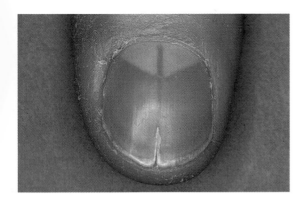

LONGITUDINAL SPLITTING OF THE NAIL

Caused by trauma with irreversible changes to the nail matrix. The present case was due to a deep needle prick in a dressmaker.

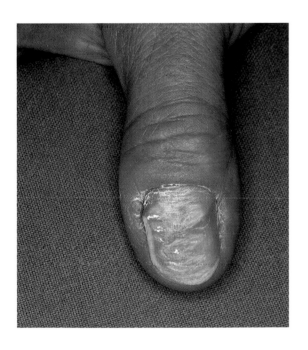

POSTTRAUMATIC ONYCHODYSTROPHY

Trauma to the fingertips can cause various types of permanent nail deformity. This case was due to a hammer blow. The tarnished nail plate is crossed by roughly parallel horizontal striae; the lunula has disappeared. The nail folds are inflamed and slightly squamous.

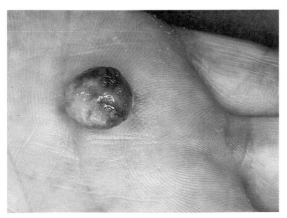

PYOGENIC GRANULOMA

A small inflammatory vascular tumor following an insect bite or other microtrauma. It begins as a small red soft fleshy mass, with no covering epidermis; it is slightly raised, and bleeds readily and profusely on contact. Older lesions gain an epidermis and undergo further vascular differentiation.

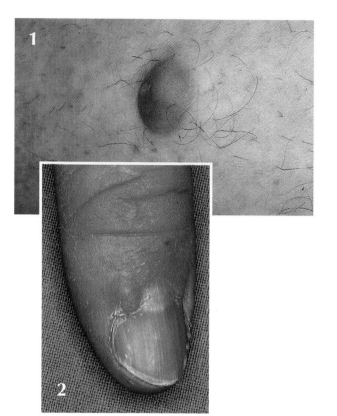

CUTANEOUS FIBROMA: ROLE OF ENVIRON-MENTAL FACTORS

A cutaneous fibroma is an intradermal nodule 5–6 mm in diameter which is firm on palpation and found generally on the lower limbs. The surface may be pigmented, smooth or slightly keratotic. It is traditionally believed to be triggered by stings and bites, particularly by insects (Photo 1). In other cases, there is documented evidence of the involvement of accidental trauma, in particular when close to the nails (Photo 2).

DOG AND CAT BITES

Bites by domestic animals, in particular dogs and cats, may sometimes display no tendency to spontaneous resolution. The illustration shows an erythemato-edematous inflammatory reaction around a crusted wound with ragged borders. The lesion requires special attention, in case of *Pasteurella multocida* infection (inoculation pasteurellosis).

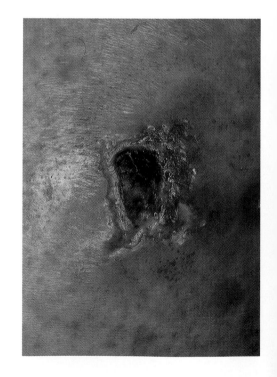

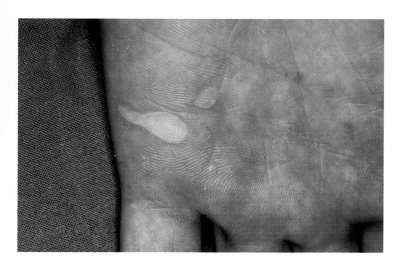

THERMAL BURNS

This elongated bulla is an occupational thermal burn of the palm caused by accidental contact during auto windshield manufacture in a glass factory.

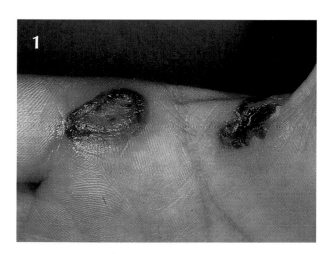

ELECTROTHERMAL BURNS

Caused by the conduction of electricity by the body (Joule effect). There is a superficial and misleading resemblance to thermal burns; the lesions are in fact deeper (Photo 1). Cure generally results in keloid scars (Photo 2).

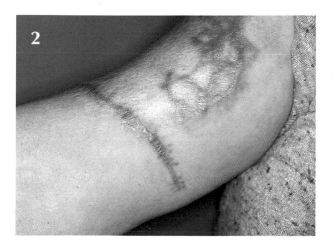

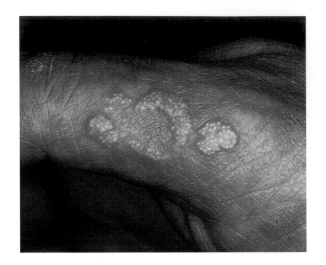

SECONDARY MILIA (RETENTION CYSTS)

Milia are superficial keratin retention cysts presenting as minute pearly, white or yellowish subepidermal inclusions 1–5 mm in diameter. They are caused by wounds or burns (as in the case illustrated) and are found mainly on the fingers and hands, where they may be either isolated or confluent. They are comparable to the milia found in some bullous diseases, in particular *epidermolysis bullosa* and *porphyria cutanea* tarda.

KELOIDS

Keloids are red prominent overgrowths of dense fibrous tissue developing over a primary lesion (wound or burn) usually several weeks after healing. They tend to be irritable and hypersensitive. They are more frequent in skin regions most subject to traction (shoulder, presternum) but may occur anywhere. The mechanism of this collagen production disorder has not been elucidated. Blacks are particularly prone to keloids perhaps because of more rapid fibroblast product turnover.

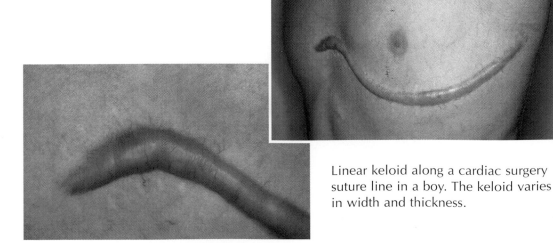

Linear keloid along a cardiac surgery suture line in a boy. The keloid varies in width and thickness.

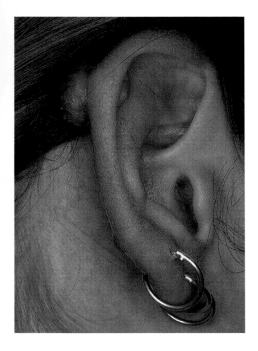

Keloid in the upper part of the pinna of the ear following the insertion of a stud ("piercing"). It is more profuse on the outer than on the inner surface where cartilage exerts greater pressure. Note the absence of a keloid reaction to the rings inserted in the ear lobe.

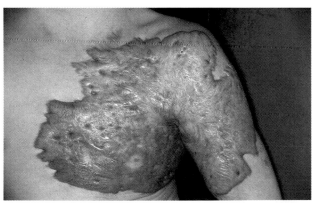

Extensive scapular keloid following a thermal burn, showing the characteristic lobster-claw borders.

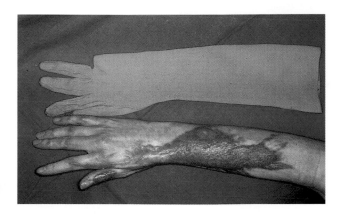

Compression therapy (using a Jobst® pressure garment) for a post-burn keloid.

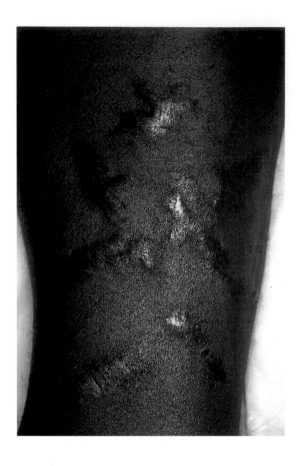

Post-trauma keloids in a Black subject.

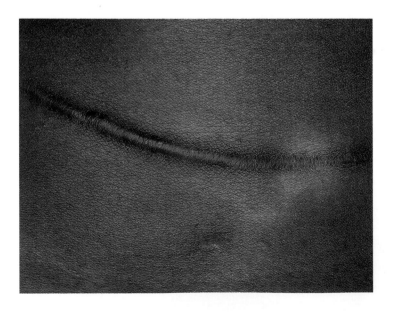

Keloid in a thyroidecto-my scar with a depig-mented plaque after ste-roid injection (a classic keloid therapy).
Post-steroid depigmenta-tion is common in Blacks.

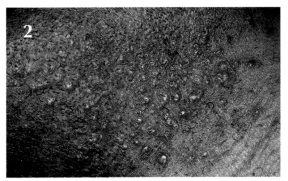

PSEUDOFOLLICULITIS BARBAE

Small inflammatory follicular papules marking a foreign body reaction to obliquely cut tightly curled hair penetrating the skin rather than passing through the follicular orifice (Photo 1). The condition is precipitated by close shaving, in particular with a single or double bladed razor, and is commoner in kinky-haired subjects (Blacks) (due to the curved follicles and the elliptic section of the hair). The deep-black inflammatory papules are generally larger than in Caucasians (Photo 2).

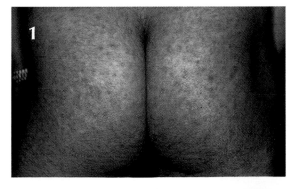

GLUTEAL PSEUDOFOLLICULITIS

As in pseudofolliculitis barbae, curvature forces the hairs into the surrounding skin after exiting from the follicles. Repeated friction is a contributory factor and the condition is particularly common in long-distance truckdrivers. The lesions are symmetrically distributed over the whole gluteal region (Photo 1) and may cause scarring (Photo 2).

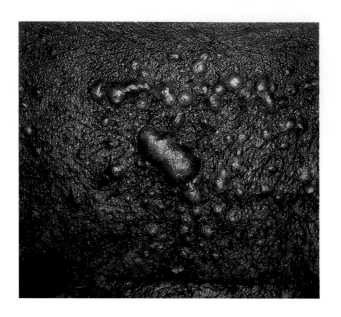

FOLLICULITIS CHELOIDALIS

This occurs only on black skin and is similar to pseudofolliculitis barbae, in that the nape of the neck hair grows into the skin, either spontaneously or after shaving. The nape of the neck is scattered with papular pseudokeloid inflammatory and/or fibrous lesions. The condition is often found in conjunction with pseudofolliculitis barbae, but not always in conjunction with acne.

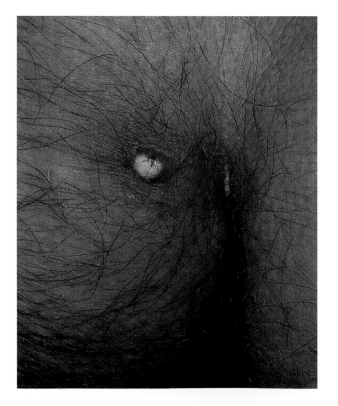

SACROCOCCYGEAL PILONIDAL CYST

Caused by the inclusion of hairs, mainly in hairy young men. The suppurating mass discharges through a fistula onto the skin. It is commonest in occupations which involve prolonged sitting: taxi drivers, truck drivers, office workers etc.

BARBER'S HAIR SINUS

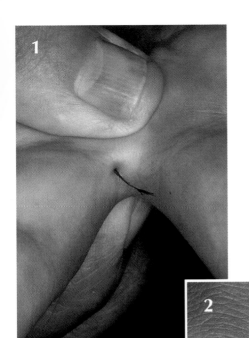

Caused by hair fragments penetrating the skin, particularly deep in the interdigital web (Photo 1), especially in the second and fourth spaces on the right hand, and more rarely on the left hand. Small purplish-red inflammatory nodules may develop, usually with an orifice in the center which discharges pus intermittently and from which hair fragments can be extracted (Photo 2).

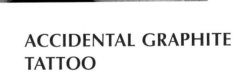

ACCIDENTAL GRAPHITE TATTOO

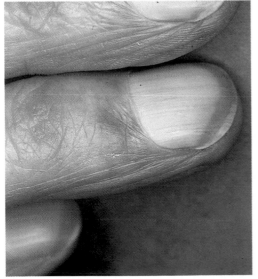

Some foreign bodies are chemically inert and hence trigger no granulomatous reaction. The classic example is accidental implantation of a pencil tip into the skin, leaving a blue-black, sometimes raised, tattoo which remains unchanged over the years. The inserted material is graphite (a hexagonal crystal carbon) which, on histology, can be seen covered in a thin fibrous capsule.

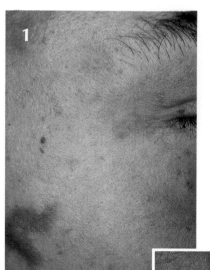

ACCIDENTAL PYROTECHNICIAN'S TATTOO

Accidental projection into the skin of red phosphorus particles on lighting firework rockets can cause blue-ish tattoos which are either punctate (Photo 1) or linear (Photo 2). The tattoo has been implanted in the nail bed (Photo 2) after phosphorus particles have traversed the nail plate. Microscopy shows necrobiotic granulomata surrounded by a giant cell palisade.

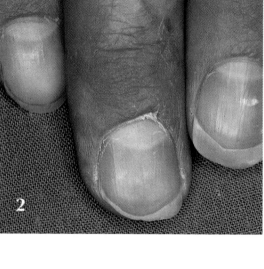

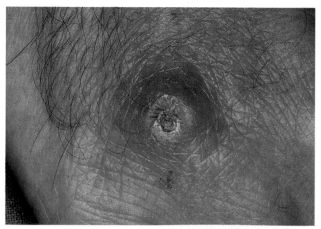

THORN INCLUSION GRANULOMA

Purplish red nodule on the dorsum of the hand in response to penetration by a rosebush thorn. The nodule has a depressed necrotic centre covered by an adherent scab. Microscopy shows a foreign body giant cell granuloma.

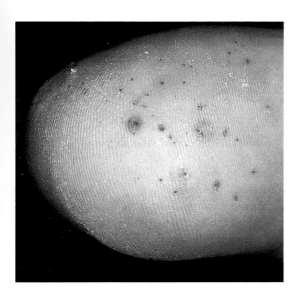

SEA URCHIN GRANULOMA

Multiple lesions on the sole of the foot caused by sea urchin spine inclusion in a barefoot holidaymaker after paddling on a rocky coastline. The spines show as black dots. Some have caused a mild erythematous reaction; others are surrounded by a greenish-blue granulomatous zone embedded in the skin. On microscopy it resembles a silica granuloma.

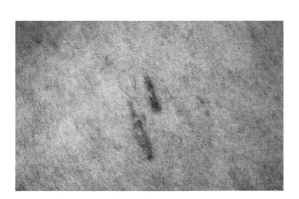

COLLIER'S STRIPES

Occupational coal dust tattoos are common in miners. They present as slate-blue linear stripes at the abrasion sites

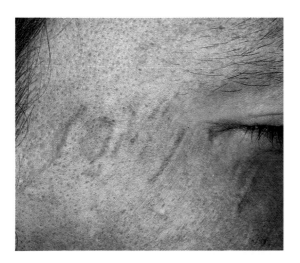

ACCIDENTAL SOIL TATTOO

Slate-blue striae in scars involving contact with the ground, caused by soil penetration of the dermis (which accounts for the blueish color).
The scars are not raised but microscopy shows mini foreign body granulomata.

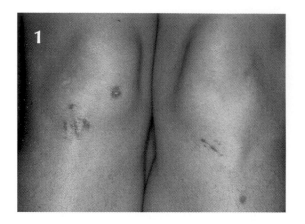

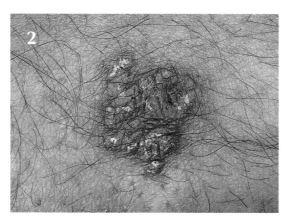

SILICA GRANULOMA

Silica granuloma is a generally painless papulonodular thickening which may be criss-crossed by purplish scars. It may develop several years after the initial accidental inoculation of silica particles into the skin. Scars at different sites are involved simultaneously (Photo 1). The scar lines may be faint, embedded in the nodular mass (Photo 2). On microscopy the lesion resembles sarcoid granuloma, which (like scar sarcoidosis) may point to systemic sarcoidosis. In silica granuloma, the reaction is a purely local immunogenic response. The delay in onset may be due to the delayed release of silica particles from the surface of the soil inclusions.

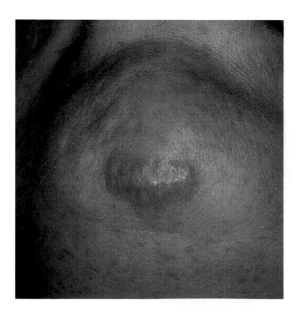

SCAR SARCOIDOSIS AS SYMPTOMATIC OF SYSTEMIC SARCOIDOSIS

An elongated purplish-red sarcoid nodule on an old chin scar. The whitish scar is clearly visible on the nodule surface, together with suture lines at right angles. This nodule was a cutaneous symptom of systemic sarcoidosis, which must always be excluded.

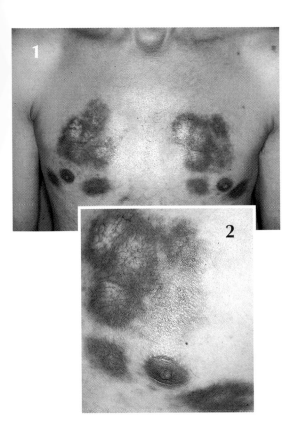

PARAFFINOMA

Caused by injecting paraffin into the dermis or subcutaneous tissue with the cosmetic aim of filling in a skin depression or highlighting an anatomical feature. This is a bodybuilder who had had paraffin injections several years earlier to enhance his apparent pectoral muscle mass (Photo 1). Sclerous lesions can be seen at the injection sites; they are golden-yellow at the center and erythematous at the periphery (Photo 2).

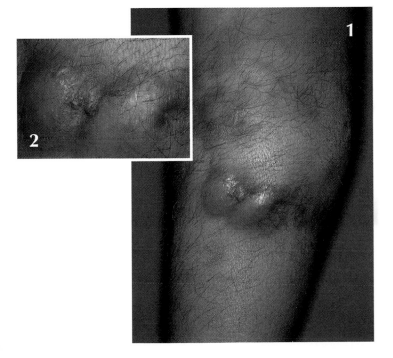

SILICONOMA

Liquid silicone may induce foreign body granulomas sometimes years after injection. In the present case, the injections had been given to reshape the calf muscles. Dark red nodules are scattered on large infiltrated sclerous plaques (Photo 1). The nodules show necrotic foci on close-up (Photo 2).

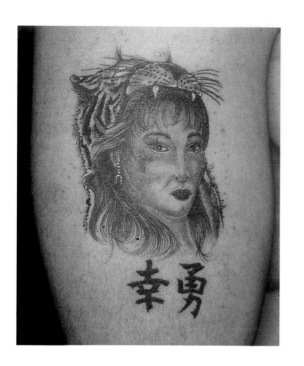

PROFESSIONAL DECORATIVE TATTOOS

This type of multicolour tattoo is performed using an electric needle which implants the insoluble pigments into the dermis at a relatively uniform depth.
The main pigments used are the following:
blue and black: carbon and Indian ink;
light blue: cobaltous aluminate;
brown: ferric oxide;
yellow: cadmium salts;
red: cinnabar (mercury-based) and plant pigments.

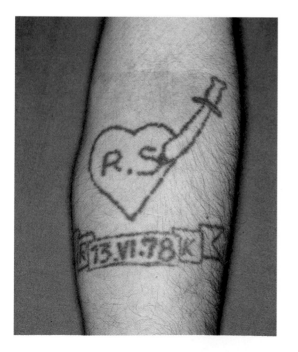

AMATEUR DECORATIVE TATTOOS

Blue-black monochrome tattoos by an amateur using a simple needle and Indian ink. Pigment depth is thus highly variable as it depends on the tattooist's dexterity and touch.
Such tattoos are typical of small closed or semi-closed communities (schools, prisons, barracks etc.) or of individuals in search of an identity.

Tattoo as a declaration of desire.

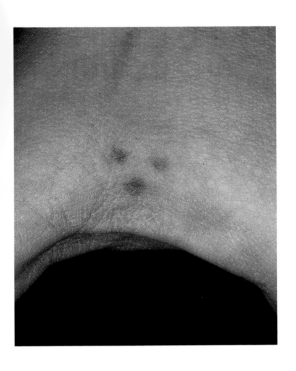

Typical closed-community (prison) tattoo. The three dots symbolize defiance.

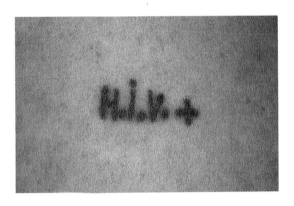

Tattoo as a badge of belonging, in this case, to the homosexual community under threat of HIV.

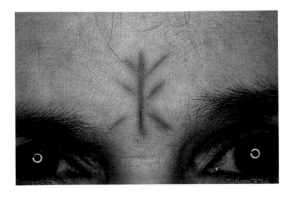

Ethnic tattoo from the Algerian coastal region bordering Morocco.

IV. OCCUPATIONAL AND LEISURE DERMATOSES OF CHEMICAL ORIGIN

CHEMICAL BURNS

The severity of chemical burns depends on:
- the type and concentration of chemical agent responsible
- duration of exposure
- other factors (occlusion, hygrometry, single or repeated exposure etc.)

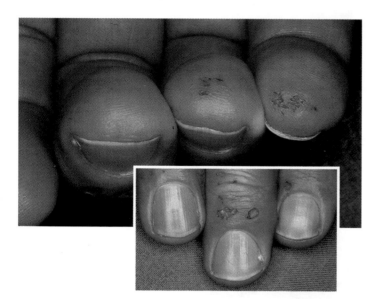

BLEACH

Painful punctate erosions of the fingertips. The repeated movements involved in stone cleaning with the bare hands accounts for the lesion topography.

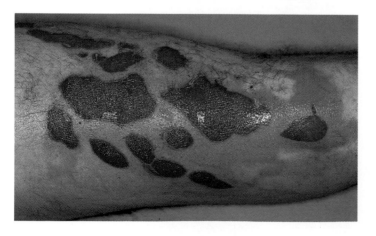

CAUSTIC SODA

Concentrated caustic soda splash on the extensor aspect of the thigh, causing superficial bullae followed by ulceration.

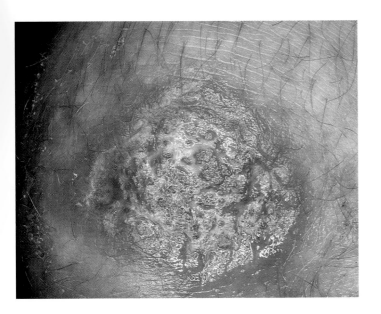

CEMENT

These are alkaline burns caused mainly but not exclusively by rapid-setting cements. The lesions are painful punched-out ulcers on the knees, anterior aspect of the legs, and feet and hands.

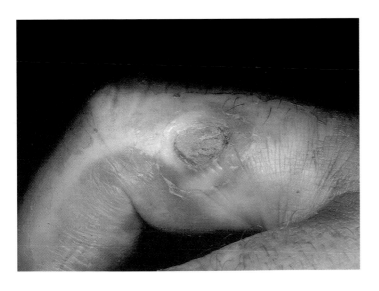

HYDROCHLORIC ACID

Acid burns are identical to alkaline burns except that healing is generally quickly. The photograph shows a punched-out necrotic finger ulcer surrounded by a large area whitened by a more superficial burn.

HYDROFLUORIC ACID

Hydrofluoric acid has a special place in occupational and leisure medicine due to the severity of the burns it causes and the specific treatment they require. It is freely available and used in the manufacture of antirust preparations.

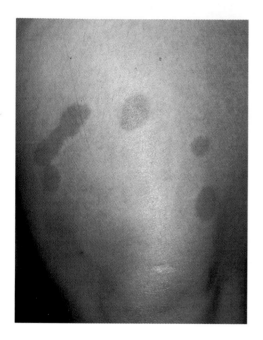

Superficial splash burn on the thigh from concentrated antirust solution. The immediate response was painful erythema, followed within hours by superficial bullae.

Deep finger pulp burn from non-perceived contact with dilute hydrofluoric acid.
The purplish burn site will inevitably progress to bulla formation and necrosis. The distinctive feature of this burn is delayed onset, several hours after contact, combined with intense pain.

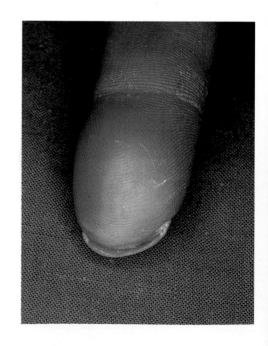

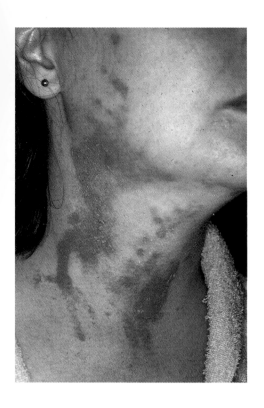

HOSPITAL ANTISEPTIC

Concentrated chlorhexidine splash burn in a female nurse, characterized by erythematous, pruritic and painful exudation on the lateral and anterior aspects of the neck and also on the face.

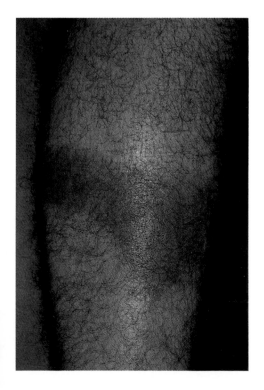

INDUSTRIAL PRESERVATIVE

Burn on the anterior and lateral aspects of the leg in a papermill worker caused by benziso-thiazolinone, a paper pulp preservative. The sharply marginated lesion was made worse by occlusion from the upper part of rubber boot.

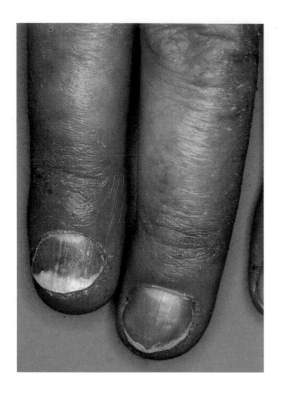

CHEMICAL LEUKONYCHIA AND ONYCHOLYSIS

Distal nail extremity in a female laboratory technician handling formalin solutions without gloves.

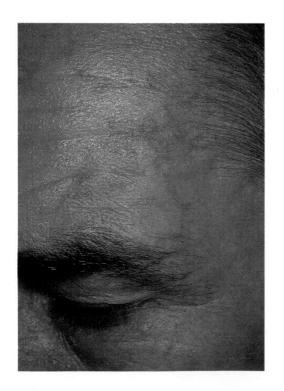

CHEMICAL HYPOMELANOSIS

Various chemical agents are melanocyto-toxic, causing often transient but sometimes permanent depigmentation, with a differential diagnosis of vitiligo.

Examples include:

para-t-butylcatechol, used as an antioxidant in various industrial processes such as plastics manufacture.

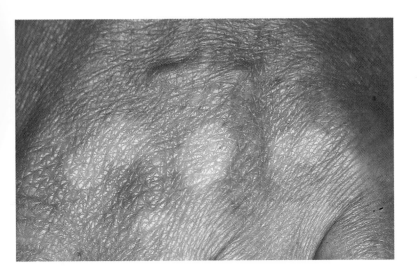

nonylphenol, used as a disinfectant, in particular in detergents.

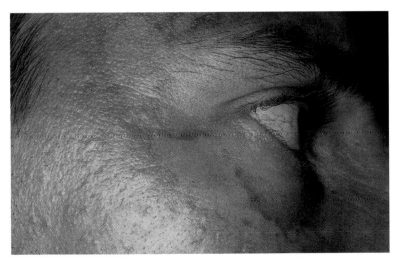

para-t-butylphenol, used as an antioxidant in rubber: the lesions mark the pressure points of a paintball helmet.

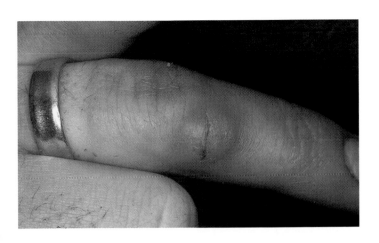

POST-TRAUMATIC MINERAL OIL GRANULOMA

Mini oiloma in a trauma wound in a metal worker in constant contact with mineral cutting oils.

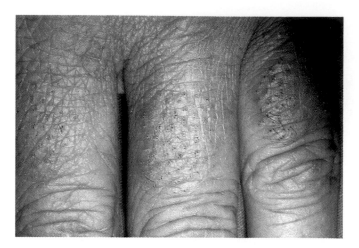

Single comedones on the back of the fingers.

OIL FOLLICULITIS

Oil folliculitis is due to exposure to industrial (mainly mineral) oils used in cutting, lubrication and cooling. Mineral oils vary in comedogenicity.

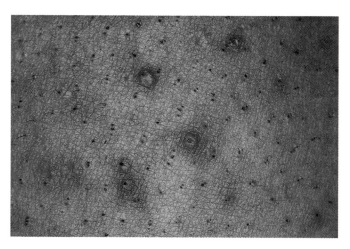

Single and double comedones and true oil spots: domed erythematous papules which are firm on palpation and topped by a single or double comedo.

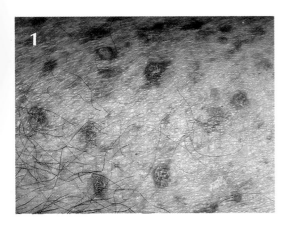

PITCH KERATOSIS

Variably sized, dirty-gray, readily bleeding keratotic papules ("pitch warts") on a poikilodermic background (irregular areas of atrophy, depigmentation, hyperpigmentation and telangiectasia) (Photos 1 and 2). Some lesions progress to true kerato-acanthomata (Photo 3), which used to be known as "pitch spots", or to squamous cell carcinoma.

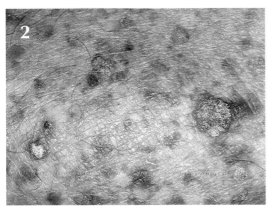

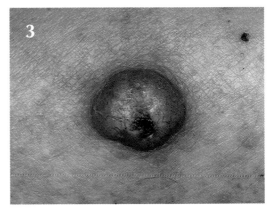

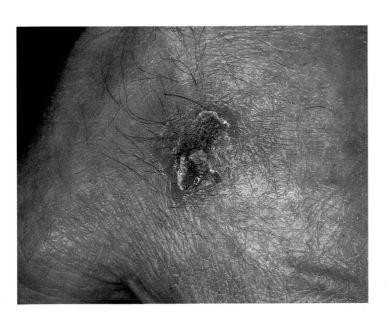

BASAL CELL CARCINOMA FOLLOWING A BURN

Basal cell carcinoma on the dorsum of the hand 3 years after a high temperature mercury splash burn in a welder.

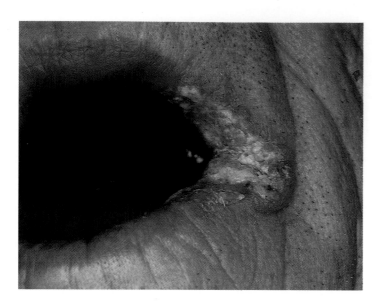

NICOTINE LEUKOPLAKIA OF THE LIP

White indurated plaque on the corner of the mouth in a pipe smoker. The raised nodular border is evidence that the lesion has transformed into a squamous cell carcinoma.

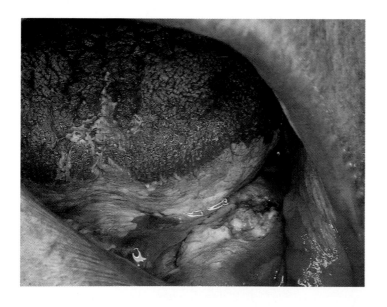

SQUAMOUS CELL CARCINOMA FOLLOWING ENDOBUCCAL NICOTINE LEUKOPLAKIA

Extensive opaline tobacco leukoplakia spreading over the tongue, palate and gums. Degeneration to squamous cell carcinoma is shown by the nodular gum ulcer.

CHEMICAL CONTACT URTICARIA

In addition to latex protein contact urticaria, illustrated in another section, many agents can cause immune and non immune urticarial reactions on direct contact with the skin.

E.g.:

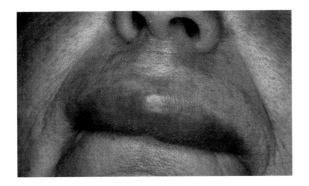

Kiwi fruit contact urticaria. This immune urticaria is triggered by proteins and in the present case has caused edematous infiltration of the upper lip.

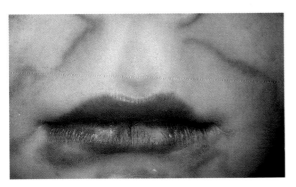

Vanilla contact urticaria in a child exposed to ice cream. The lesions extend not only to the lips but also to the perioral area.

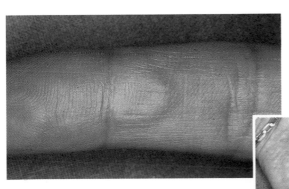

Plant contact urticaria. Non immune contact urticaria of the fingers in a flower arranger after handling *Heliopsis scarbra*.

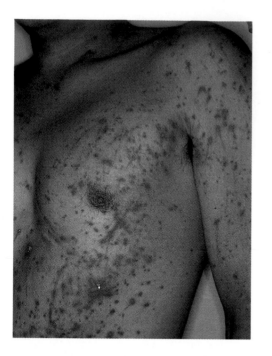

PHYTOPHOTODERMATITIS (MEADOW DERMATITIS)

An erythemato-vesicular or bullous photo-toxic eruption at the points of skin contact with a plant. The dermatosis is produced by a combination of three factors: sun, humidity and plant contact.

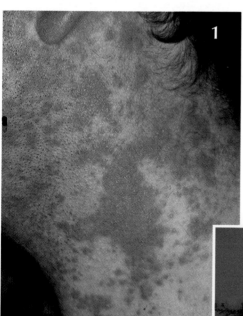

AIRBORNE CONTACT DERMATITIS: FRULLANIA

Hand- and airborne contact dermatitis (Photo 1) to *Frullania dilatata* (Photo 2) in a forestry worker. *Frullania* is a liverwort which grows on tree trunks and branches (oak, beech, acacia, poplar etc) and rocks.
The allergen is (+) frullanolide, a sesquiterpene lactone.

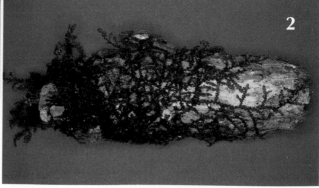

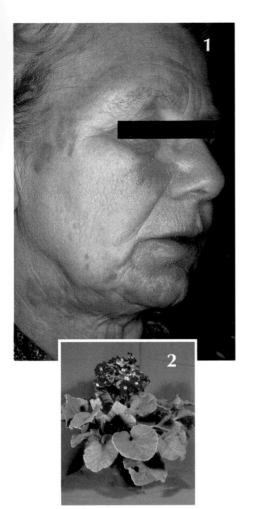

ALLERGIC CONTACT DERMATITIS: PRIMROSE

Allergic contact dermatitis (Photo 1) to *Primula obconica* (Photo 2). The lesions are handborne and in the present case affect the temples, cheeks, chin and neck.

The most important allergen is primine, a quinone present in the plant at peak concentrations between April and August.

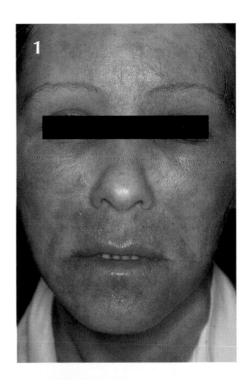

ALLERGIC CONTACT DERMATITIS: ALSTROEMERIA

Occupational allergic contact dermatitis in a female florist (Photo 1) after handling Alstroemeria (Photo 2). The eruption is both hand- and airborne.

One of the allergens is tuliposide A (also responsible for tulip finger).

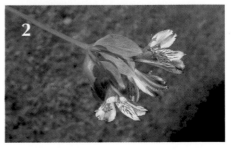

83

FIBREGLASS DERMATITIS

Fibreglass dermatitis covers all the clinical manifestations of contact with glass silk, glass wool, and rock wool. The lesions are hand- and/or airborne. Identical milder lesions are caused by other fibrous materials: cellulose, cardboard, mica, polypropylene, carbon etc. The main symptom is intense pruritus and the main sign is punctate excoriation due to direct penetration of fibres (4–20 μm in diameter) into the epidermis.

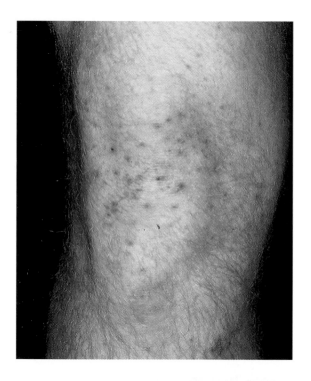

Punctate erosions of the knee.

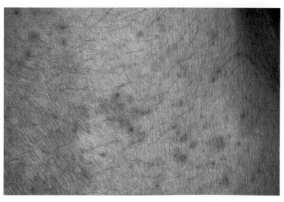

Erosions on the dorsum of the hand. Each erosion is surrounded by a highly inflammatory micropapule.

AIRBORNE FUME IRRITANT DERMATITIS

Fumes cause airborne irritant dermatitis usually involving the face.

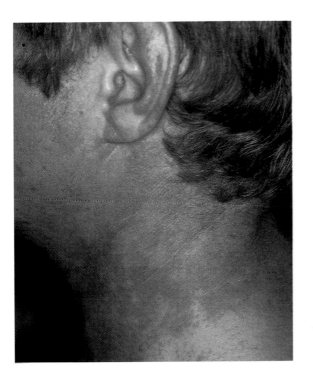

Perchlorethylene fume irritant dermatitis after cleaning an unventilated tank. Extensive, erythematous, pruritic and slightly painful plaques on the lateral aspect of the neck.

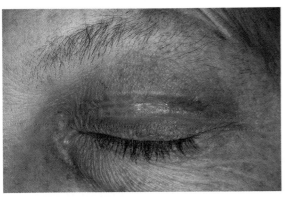

Formalin fume irritant dermatitis due to unprotected plastic goods manufacture. Extensive, erythematous, edematous and erosive blepharitis was associated with burning pains. The formalin patch test was negative.

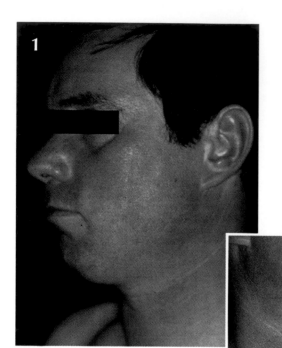

AIRBORNE PHOTOTOXIC TAR CONTACT DERMATITIS

Extensive erythematous eruption on the face (Photo 1) and neck (Photo 2) in an asphalt worker. Other tars, e.g. bitumen, pitch, creosote and coal tar, may cause similar airborne eruptions.

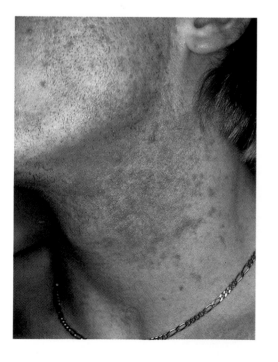

AIRBORNE ALLERGIC CONTACT DERMATITIS

The signs are those of typical allergic contact dermatitis; the lesions are symmetrical in most cases. They can be acute or chronic, depending on the modalities of onset (type and/or concentration of allergen, frequency of airborne contact etc).
Lesion distribution is typical. Exposed areas – face, neck, neckline – are most often involved.

Airborne dermatitis: cement dust. Pruritic erythematous vesicular lesions of the face and neck. The potassium dichromate patch test was positive.

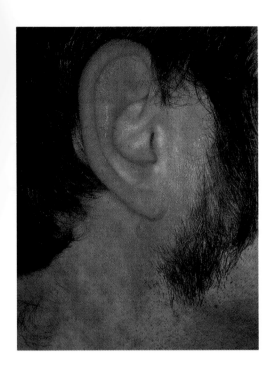

Airborne dermatitis: epoxy resin. Pruritic erythematous edematous lesions on the lateral aspects of the neck. The epoxy resin patch test was positive.

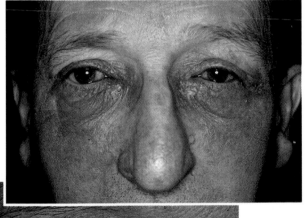

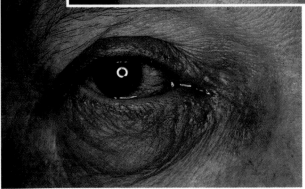

Airborne dermatitis: powdered pig feed. Acute symmetrical and intensely pruritic blepharo-conjunctivitis. The patch test to olaquindox (an antiseptic and growth promoting piglet feed additive) was positive.

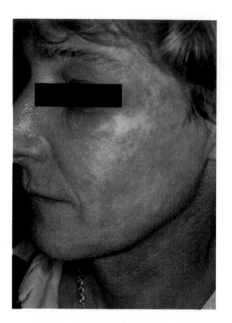

Airborne dermatitis: propacetamol (Pro-Dafalgan®), in a female nurse splashed prior to injection into the infusion set. Erythematous intensely pruritic lesions of the face and neck, with marked malar edema. The propacetamol patch test was positive; the paracetamol patch test was negative.

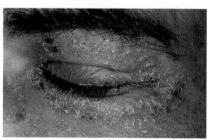

Airborne dermatitis: cephalosporin for injection, in a male nurse. Excoriated erythemato-squamous lesions of the eyelids. The cefotaxime patch test was positive.

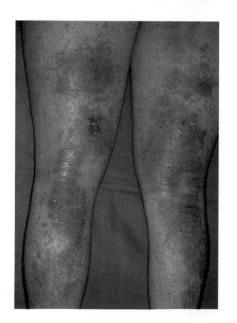

ALLERGIC CONTACT DERMATITIS: IMITATION LEATHER DYE

Acute erosive exudative dermatitis confined to the posterior aspect of the lower limbs after prolonged contact with brown imitation chair leather.
The Disperse Yellow 3 patch test was positive.

V. DERMATOSES CAUSED BY MEDICAL MATERIALS

ALLERGIC CONTACT DERMATITIS: SURGICAL TAPE

Allergic contact dermatitis to various surgical adhesive tapes is well recognized. Traditional surgical tapes contain colophony gum, whereas the more modern paper tapes use acrylic resins and are less frequently involved.

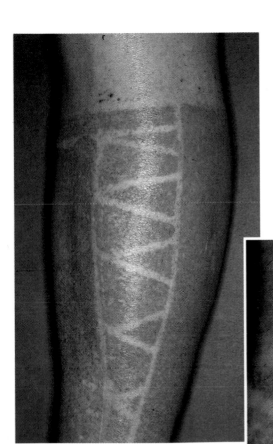

Contact dermatitis to an adhesive limb strapping used in sports medicine. Erythemato-edematous eczema is confined to the area of adhesive application, and does not affect the linear areas covered by the intersecting fabric tape between the skin and the strapping. The colophony patch test was positive.

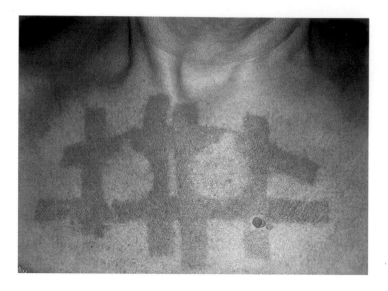

Contact dermatitis to an adhesive tape used to secure electrocardiograph electrodes to the skin. The eczema is confined to the areas where the strips of tape were applied, i.e. the sites of electrode application are unaffected, as is the surround of a small melanotic naevus. The ethylhexylacrylate patch test was positive.

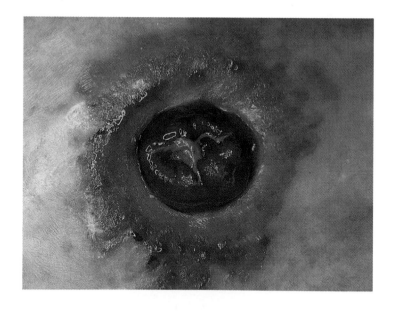

ALLERGIC CONTACT DERMATITIS: STOMA POUCH

Plaque of peristomal allergic contact dermatitis to a self-adhesive stoma pouch incorporating a karaya gum skin protector. The erythro-vesicular lesion is scattered with erosions and its margins are ill-defined. The karaya gum patch test was positive.

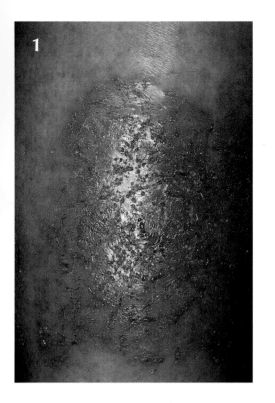

ALLERGIC CONTACT DERMATITIS: HYDROCOLLOID DRESSING

A rare reaction seen with dressings containing a colophony derivative. In this case, the dressing had been applied to an ulcer during epidermis formation (Photo 1). The reaction is an extensive and partially ulcerating erythrovesicular plaque (Photo 2). The colophony patch test was positive.

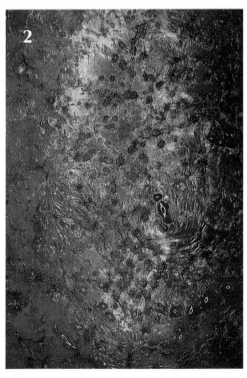

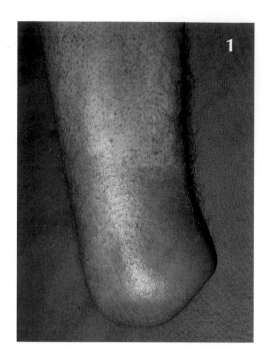

INTOLERANCE TO PROSTHESES AND ORTHOSES

Devices in contact with the skin can cause intolerance, the prime example being the orthopedic appliances fitted to amputation stumps. If ill-fitting, they cause friction dermatosis (Photo 1). They can also cause allergic contact dermatitis to a chemical constituent of the device in direct contact with the skin – in this case, to a rubberized internal support (Photo 2). The Mercapto Mix patch test was positive.

Allergic contact dermatitis to the dyes and plastics used in orthoses is becoming increasingly common.

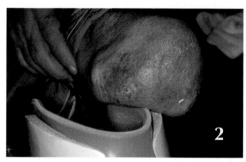

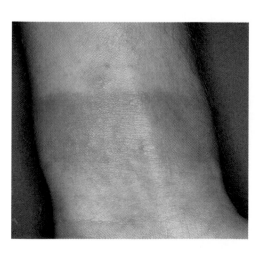

ALLERGIC CONTACT DERMATITIS: SURGICAL GLOVES

Surgical latex gloves may cause allergic contact dermatitis to various additives, in particular those that accelerate vulcanization. This sharply marginated erythemato-edematous plaque occurred on the flexor aspect of the forearm in a female anesthetist.

The Thiuram Mix patch test was positive.

IMMUNE CONTACT URTICARIA: LATEX GLOVES

Immune contact urticaria to latex surgical gloves has become a major problem in environmental dermatology, with a dramatic increase in incidence following the introduction of new latex processing techniques releasing various proteins with molecular weights ranging from 2 to 30 kiloDaltons. These proteins penetrate intact skin and induce immediate urticarial allergic reactions mediated by immunoglobulin E. Powdered gloves are particularly responsible in that the cornstarch concentrates the latex proteins. Starch is so volatile that in hospitals, and especially operating theatres, airborne urticaria is seen in highly sensitized subjects even if they themselves are not wearing the gloves in question.

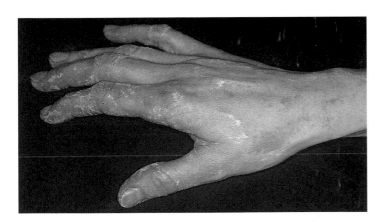

Immune contact urticaria of the hands from internally powdered latex gloves. The dorsa show erythematous plaques dotted with small urticarial papules.

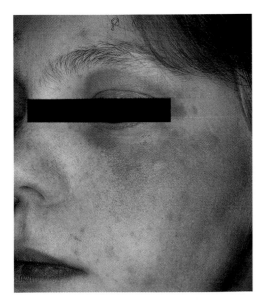

Airborne immune contact urticaria of the face caused by the dispersion of cornstarch particles with a high latex protein content in a female operating theatre nurse presensitized by latex gloves. Urticarial plaques on the cheeks, eyelids and nostril areas, associated with conjunctivitis and allergic rhinitis.

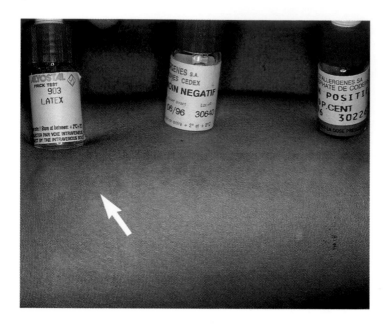

Prick test with commercial latex (Stallergènes®). The latex prick test (left of illustration) is strongly positive, causing an urticarial reaction surrounded by an erythematous ring. The codeine sulfate prick test (positive control : right of illustration) shows a less marked urticarial reaction while the prick test with normal saline (negative control: center of illustration) shows no reaction.

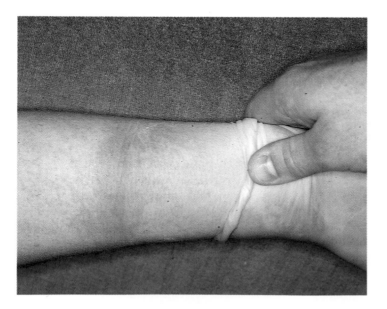

Positive challenge test with a latex glove in a presensitized individual, showing a vast urticarial plaque.

VI. DERMATOSES CAUSED BY CLOTHES AND CLOTHING ACCESSORIES

ALLERGIC CONTACT DERMATITIS: SHOES

Allergic contact dermatitis to shoes has become a major problem. The most frequently reported allergens are chromium salts (leather tanning agents), formaldehyde paratertiary butylphenol resin (used as a glue), rubber additives, and dyes,

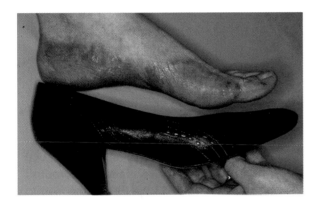

Allergic contact dermatitis to a glue used in shoe manufacture. The topography of the mildly edematous, erythemato-squamous eczema is highly typical. The formaldehyde paratertiary butylphenol resin patch test was positive.

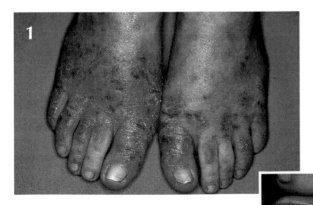

Allergic contact dermatitis to a leather shoe, typically confined to the dorsum of the foot and toes with no extension to the interdigital webs (Photo 2), showing crusty fissured erythema (Photo 3). The potassium dichromate patch test was positive.

ALLERGIC CONTACT DERMATITIS: RUBBERIZED CLOTHING

Rubberized garments are common sources of allergic contact dermatitis; the primary allergens are agents that accelerate vulcanization.

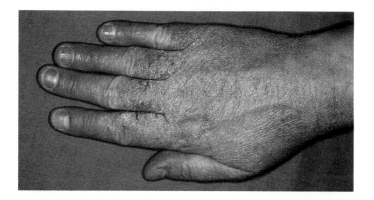

Allergic contact dermatitis to a household rubber glove. Dry fissured erythemato-squamous hyperkeratosis on the dorsa of the hands. The Thiuram Mix patch test was positive.

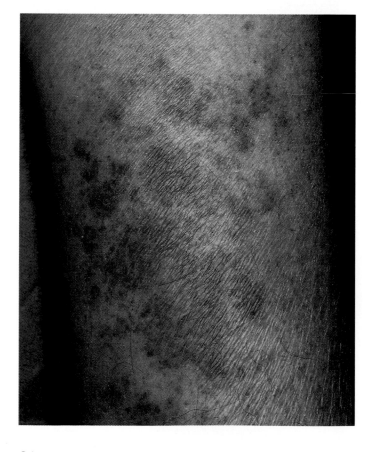

Allergic contact dermatitis to a rubber boot. The lesions are distinctive in being not simply erythemato-vesicular but also markedly purpuric, as is frequent on the lower limbs. The Mercapto Mix patch test was positive.

ALLERGIC CONTACT DERMATITIS: CLOTHING FABRIC

Clothing fabrics, whether made of natural or artificial fibres, cause an allergic contact dermatitis which in some cases can be diagnosed simply from its topography. The two main allergens are various synthetic fibre constituents and dyes.

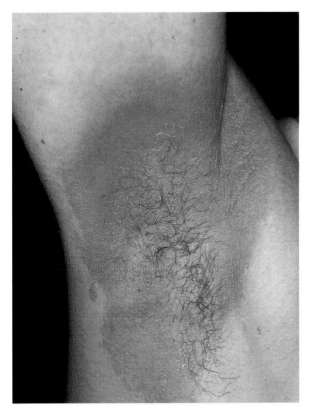

Allergic contact dermatitis to the dye in a blue dress. Allergen dissolution by sweat accounts for the axillary location. Mildly infiltrated erythematous eczema involves the entire axilla except deep in the fold, where the allergen is probably more dilute. The Disperse Blue 106 patch test was positive.

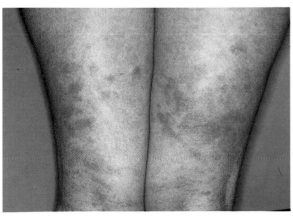

Allergic contact dermatitis to a diving suit, typically localized to the posterior aspect of the thighs due to greater suit-skin friction in this area. Atopic dermatitis may be a differential diagnosis in some cases. The paraphenylenediamine and Disperse Yellow 3 patch tests were positive.

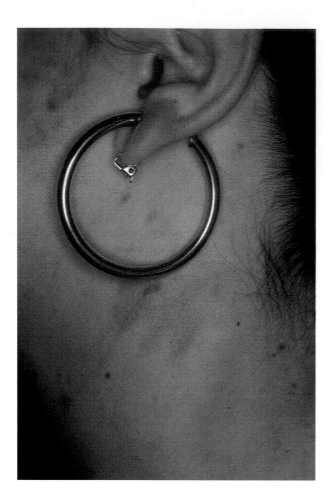

ALLERGIC CONTACT DERMATITIS: NICKEL

Nickel is the most common environmental contact allergen: in the industrialized world, approximately 10 % of adult women are sensitized; the figures reported for men are much lower, but vary between studies. The reason for the sex difference is ear piercing in girls, which induces the allergy. Earrings (unless in yellow gold or platinum) are responsible for most contact dermatitis but the diversity of clinical sites reflects the range of nickel-releasing clothing accessories also involved: jean studs, watch strap clips, necklaces, bracelets, suspenders, metal shoe eyes etc. Dermatologists disagree over the role of coins in exacerbating hand eczema in subjects allergic to nickel. The question remains unresolved. The European Union has decided to refrain the use of nickel in the coins of the forthcoming single currency (Euro).

Allergic contact dermatitis to an earring, showing red edema of the earlobe and erythematous plaques on the lateral aspect of the neck due to repeated rubbing by the ring. The nickel sulfate patch test was positive.

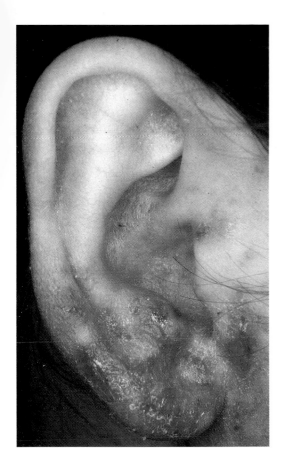

Allergic contact dermatitis to a clip-on earring : crusty exudative erythema of the lobe and lower pinna. The nickel sulfate patch test was positive.

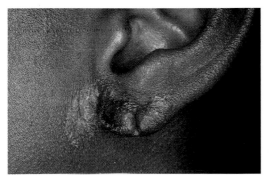

Allergic contact dermatitis to an earring in an African woman. The lesion is granulomatous because the earrings continued to be worn despite the eczematous reaction. The nickel sulfate patch test was positive.

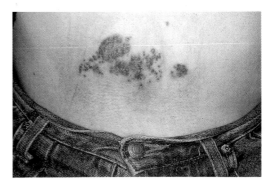

Allergic contact dermatitis to a jean stud, extending far beyond the friction area. The nickel sulfate patch test was positive.

VII. COSMETIC DERMATOSES

The cosmetic industry is undergoing exponential growth and diversification, with products targeted at aging skin, dry skin, acne, seborrhea etc. Cosmetics are used mainly for the embellishment of the skin and the reduction or camouflage of certain imperfections, thus allowing an individual's social or professional integration. Cosmetics are becoming increasingly active and effective, blurring the boundary with pharmaceuticals, and creating a new entity – cosmeceuticals – for agents that are neither simple cosmetics nor fully fledged drugs (retinoic acid, hydroquinone etc).

Cosmetics cause a variety of side effects despite an increased concern to produce formulations that are well-tolerated and minimally allergenic.

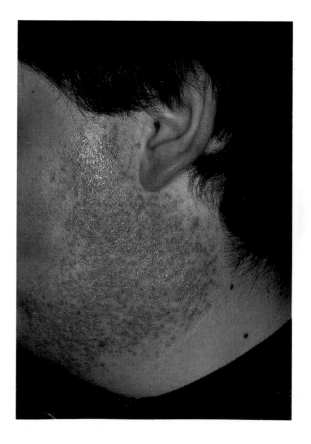

ALLERGIC CONTACT DERMATITIS: AFTERSHAVE

Acute extensive vesicular eczema stretching across the entire cheek to the earlobe after a few applications of aftershave. The Fragrance Mix and individual constituent patch tests were negative. The repeated open application test (ROAT) with the aftershave on the flexor aspect of the forearm was positive after four applications.

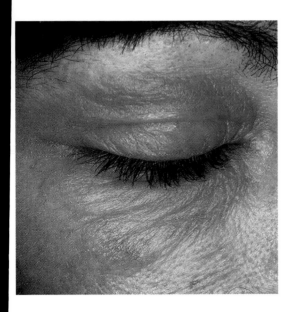

ALLERGIC CONTACT DERMATITIS: FACE CREAM

Extensive erythemato-edematous plaque with scattered vesicles over the upper and lower eyelids, with fairly distinct margins, 2 weeks after daily application of a face cream. The patch test to the preservative, imidazolidinylurea, was positive. Confinement of the lesion to the eye lids, without involving the cheeks or forehead, is explained by the specific features of the stratum corneum of the eyelid epidermis, which allows greater penetration by allergens than does the surrounding skin.

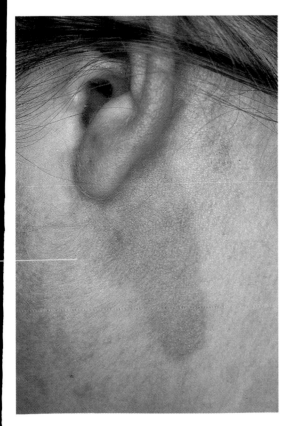

ALLERGIC CONTACT DERMATITIS: PERFUME

A sharply marginated oblong erythematous plaque on the neck below the retroauricular groove, after dabbing with a few drops of perfume. The plaque follows the perfume track [as in "berloque" – properly, breloque (modern French – pendant) dermatitis]. Positive Fragrance Mix patch test, and positive ROAT with the perfume on the flexor aspect of the forearm.

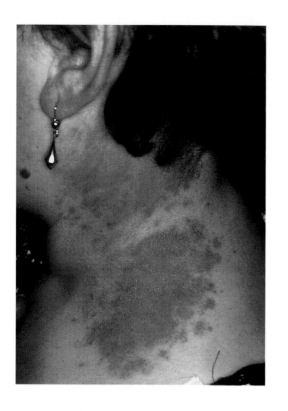

ALLERGIC CONTACT DERMATITIS: HAIR DYE

Extensive erythemato-vesicular eczema with ragged ill-defined margins on the lateral aspect of the neck, 24 hours after a perm and dye. The scalp is erythematous and extremely pruritic. The patch test to the hair dye constituent, paraphenylenediamine, was positive.

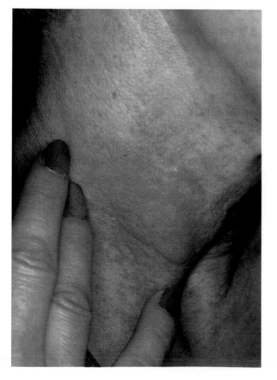

ALLERGIC CONTACT DERMATITIS: NAIL VARNISH

Poorly demarcated eczematous erythema-to-edematous plaque with ill-defined borders on the lateral aspect of the neck. Nail varnish was the likely cause in this case: the patch test with toluene sulfonamide formaldehyde resin was positive. This is a classic instance of "ectopic" or "transfer" allergic contact dermatitis, with the allergen having been transferred by the fingernails to a skin region where it was not meant to be applied. This is also known as handborne dermatitis. Careful examination showed mild periungual eczema.
The lesions fully resolved after the withdrawal of the nail varnish.

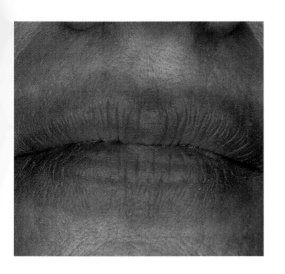

ALLERGIC CONTACT CHEILITIS AND PERICHEILITIS DUE TO A LIP PENCIL

Reaction to several applications of a lip pencil balm supposedly cicatrising and used in this case for dry lips. The balsam of Peru patch test was positive. Similar reactions occur to sunscreen pencils and lip-stick, involving a wide variety of allergens.

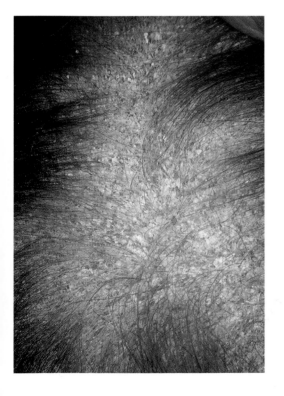

RESIDUAL DANDRUFF AFTER ALLERGIC CONTACT DERMATITIS

The distinctive feature of allergic contact dermatitis of the scalp is that dandruff, which may be truly squamous in some cases, persists after contact has ceased. It improves gradually over several weeks with appropriate treatment. In the present case, a conditioner was the probable culprit. Positive conditioner open test, but the allergen could not be identified due to lack of information. The case illustrates the importance of comprehensive package labelling of cosmetics.

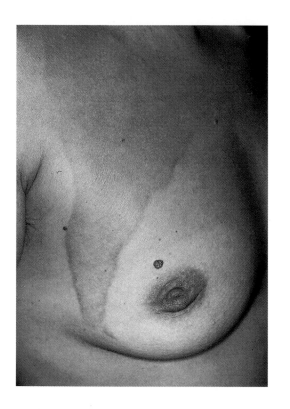

BERLOQUE DERMATITIS

A phototoxic reaction to a perfume, with two determinants: application of a perfume, followed by exposure to sunlight or (sunbed) UVR. The acute phototoxic reaction is mild but hyperpigmentation subsequently develops along the perfume track, and is exacerbated by further exposure. The case illustrated is highly typical : brown pigmentation extending over the lateral aspect of the face and chest, with a sharp hyperpigmented margin reflecting the higher perfume concentration at this point in its flow.

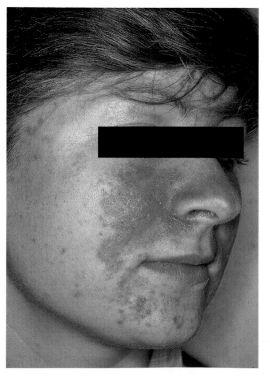

SEBORRHEIC DERMATITIS EXACERBATED BY FACE CREAM

Florid facial seborrheic dermatitis extending not only to the ala nasi but also to the cheeks, chin, forehead and temples, following repeated application of a moisturizing cream. The facial skin of subjects with seborrheic dermatitis is particularly irritable and the application of various cosmetic products which are well-tolerated by a normal skin can exacerbate the condition. The photograph depicts the conjunction of underlying seborrheic dermatitis with an irritation dermatitis caused by the cosmetic.

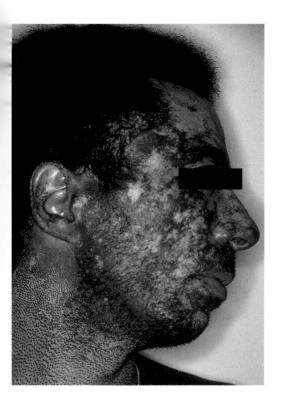

HYPOMELANOCYTIC LEUKODERMA INDUCED BY HYDROQUINONE MONO-BENZYLETHER

Variably sized patches of facial hypomela-nocytosis in a dark-skinned Sahel African due to repeated application of a "skin whitening" cream containing the melanocyto-toxic agent, hydroquinone monobenzyl-ether. Such a dramatic effect is not unusual. Repigmentation took place gradually over the ensuing months.

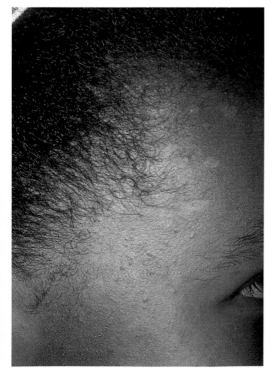

TRACTION ALOPECIA

Traction alopecia on the temples of a Black woman, as often observed in association with hair straightening, braids, tight pony tails, curlers and perms. In the present case it is combined with evidence of hypomela-nocytosis caused by a "skin whitening" cream containing hydroquinone.

FACIAL ACNE CAUSED BY COSMETICS

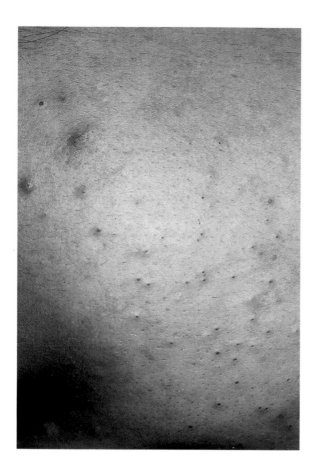

Cosmetic-induced facial acne showing crops of open black comedones and some papulo-pustules following the use of a oily cream in the evenings. Comedo acne has become rarer now that the raw materials used in cosmetics are better selected and that most oil-based cosmetics are pretested for comedogenicity.

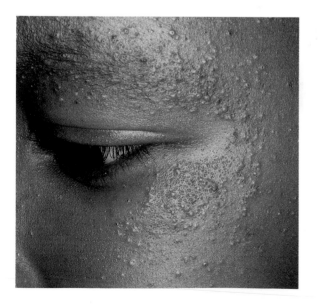

Cosmetic-induced facial acne in a young African woman after repeated application of creams containing concentrated vegetable oils and semi-fluid paraffin (vaseline). The clinical picture is characteristic, with crops of closed comedones (microcysts) scattered over the cheeks and temples, extending to the eyebrows. The eyelids are not involved, due to the absence of sebaceous follicles on the eyelid skin.

SCALP GRANULOMA FOLLOWING THE REJECTION OF ARTIFICIAL HAIR IMPLANTS

Rejection of a synthetic hair implant for male baldness.

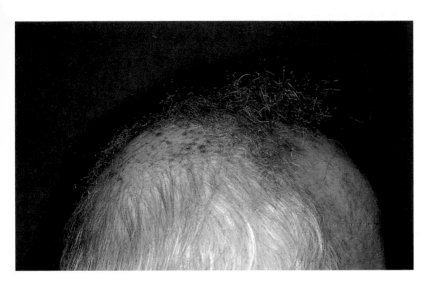

General view of the area of vertex alopecia where the artificial hair implant had been performed.

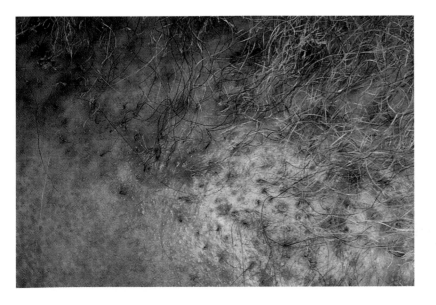

Close-up showing the loss of many implanted hairs and the presence of small rejection granulomas, characterized by an erythematous inflammatory reaction at each implantation site, with multiple crusts.

VIII. DRUG-INDUCED DERMATOSES

CUTANEOUS REACTIONS TO SYSTEMICALLY ADMINISTERED DRUGS

NON IMMUNE DRUG-INDUCED URTICARIA

Example chosen : **ACETYLSALICYLIC ACID (aspirin)**

Urticarial papules progressing from hour to hour 36 hours after exposure. Challenge can trigger the lesions within minutes.
Acetylsalicylic acid urticaria is a classic example of non immune urticaria (direct release of mast cell histamine).

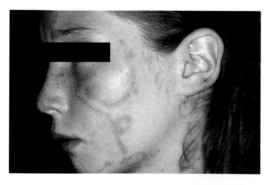

Circinate lesions are typical of drug-induced urticaria in children.

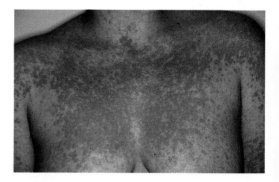

In adults, the lesions are often arranged in symmetrical sheets, with no circinate pattern.

Non immune urticaria: main drugs responsible

- Acetylsalicylic acid
- Codeine
- Contrast agents
- General anesthetics
- Hydralazine
- Nonsteroidal antiinflammatory drugs

IMMUNE DRUG-INDUCED URTICARIA

Example chosen: **AMOXICILLIN**

Extensive plaques of symmetrical highly pruritic urticaria 12–24 hours after exposure.
This is an example of IgE-dependent (type 1) immune urticaria associated with intense pruritus. The patient is afebrile.
Investigations may include prick tests with penicillin (major and minor determinants).
Reintroduction may be attempted (a single 500 mg dose), except if the reaction is severe.

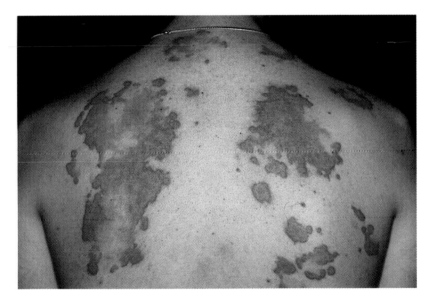

Immune urticaria: main drugs responsible
- Amoxicillin
- Ampicillin
- Cefaclor

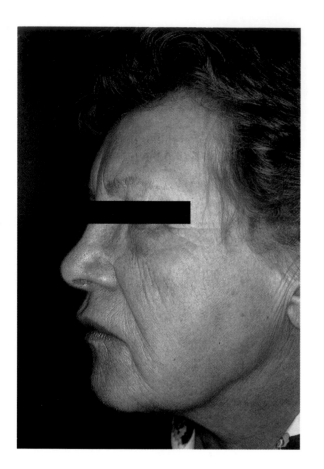

DRUG-INDUCED FACIAL ANGIOEDEMA

Example chosen: **ANGIOTENSIN CONVERTING ENZYME INHIBITOR**

Deep skin-coloured papules causing substantial swelling of the face and lips in particular. The prognosis may be guarded, particularly in the presence of concomitant involvement of the glottis and/or epiglottis.

Angioedema: main drugs responsible

- Acetylsalicylic acid
- Angiotensin converting enzyme inhibitors
- Indomethacin
- Streptokinase
- Sumatriptan

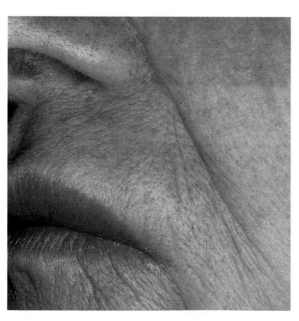

DRUG-INDUCED PSEUDO SERUM SICKNESS

Example chosen : **CEFACLOR**

Combined urticaria and angioedema seen mainly in infants below 5 years of age between 5 days and 3 weeks after initial exposure. The urticaria is often figurate or polycyclic. Associated signs and symptoms include severe joint pain, fever, lymphadenopathy and proteinuria. Dermographism may also be present. The reaction may also occur in the absence of prior exposure. Reintroduction must on no account be attempted.

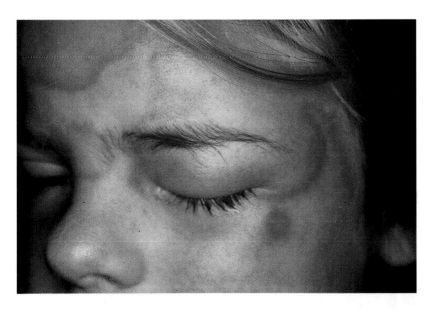

Pseudo serum sickness: main drugs responsible

- Cefaclor
- Minocyclin

DRUG-INDUCED MACULOPAPULAR RASH

Example chosen : **AMPICILLIN**

A symmetrical pruritic maculopapular rash resembling rubella (Photo 1), measles (Photo 2) or scarlet fever. In the latter case, it may progress to authentic desquamatory erythroderma (Photos 3 & 4) with some purpuric features.

The pruritus is moderate to severe. Low grade eosinophilia is often present. Rash onset is between a few and 10–15 days after initial exposure. Delayed onset (up to 2 weeks after discontinuation) is typical with penicillins. In the absence of alternative therapy (i.e. if the drug is absolutely essential), cautious reintroduction can be attempted.

A differential diagnosis of viral infection must always be borne in mind: signs in favor include lymphadenopathy, fever and conjunctivitis.

Drug-induced maculopapular rash: main drugs responsible

- Ampicillin
- Carbamazepine
- Cephalosporins
- Hydantoins
- Isoniazid
- Meprobamate
- Nonsteroidal antiinflamma-
  tory drugs
- Penicillins
- Sulfonamide antibacterials
- Sulfonamide diuretics
- Sulfonylureas

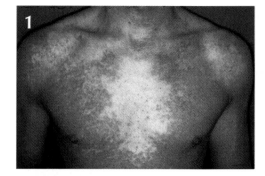

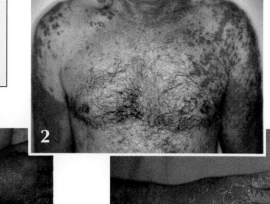

HYPERSENSITIVITY SYNDROME

Example chosen : **ALLOPURINOL**

Papular erythemato-purplish hypersensitivity rash spreading rapidly over the entire skin surface, on average 4–8 weeks after exposure. The major concomitant signs are fever, lymphadenopathy, hepatitis, neuritis, pneumonia and agranulocytosis.

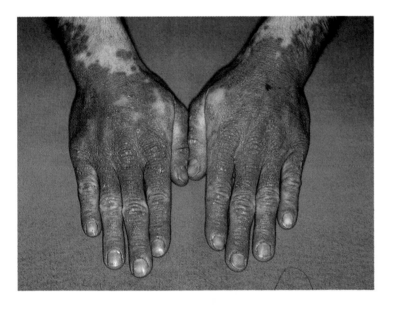

Hypersensitivity syndrome: main drugs responsible

- Allopurinol
- Carbamazepine
- Hydantoins
- Nonsteroidal antiinflammatory drugs (especially piroxicam)
- Phenobarbital
- Sulfonamide antibacterials (sulfamethoxazole)
- Sulfones

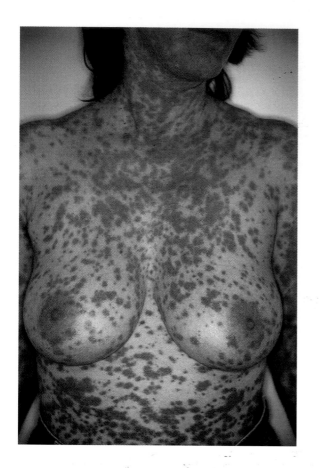

DRUG-INDUCED PURPURA

Example chosen : **ISONIAZID**

Purpuric macular rash with or without thrombocytopenia (vascular purpura or thrombocytopenic purpura). The drugs responsible may often cause both types of purpura. Note that all drug-induced rashes may be associated with some purpuric lesions. Reintroduction may be attempted in absolute necessity, providing both patch and *in-vitro* specific antibody tests are negative.

Drug-induced purpura: main drugs responsible

- Acetylsalicylic acid
- Allopurinol
- Beta-blockers
- Chlorothiazide
- Cytostatics
- Isoniazid
- Methyldopa
- Nonsteroidal antiinflammatory drugs
- Quinolones
- Valproate

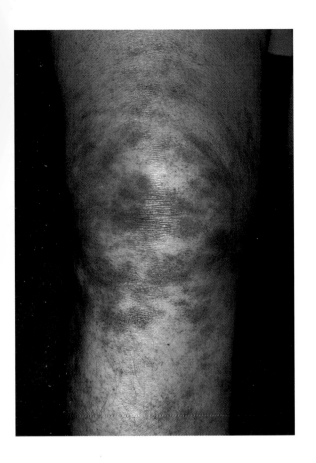

CAPILLARITIS WITH A PURPURIC AND PIGMENTED RASH

Example chosen: **CARBROMAL**

Purpuric, latterly brownish macules, non pruritic, symmetrical and poorly demarcated, found mainly on the lower limbs.

Capillaritis with a purpuric and pigmented rash: main drugs responsible

- Carbamazepine
- Carbromal
- Meprobamate

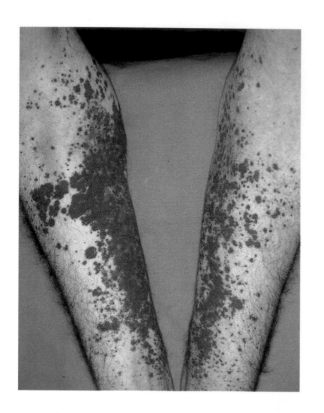

DRUG-INDUCED VASCULITIS

Example chosen: **QUINOLONE**

Symmetrical palpable purpura usually on the lower and upper limbs. Drug-induced vasculitis generally begins as a nonspecific erythemato-macular rash giving way to fully purpuric papules. There may also be hemorrhagic bullae, which may ulcerate.

The histology is often highly characteristic, showing lymphocytic or, more commonly, leukocytoclastic vasculitis with fibrinoid degeneration.

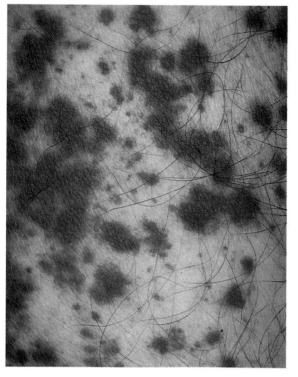

Vasculitis:
main drugs responsible
- Ampicillin
- Angiotensin converting enzyme inhibitors
- Cimetidine
- Hydantoins
- Nonsteroidal antiinflammatory drugs
- Propylthiouracil
- Quinolones
- Ranitidine
- Sulfonamides
- Thiazides

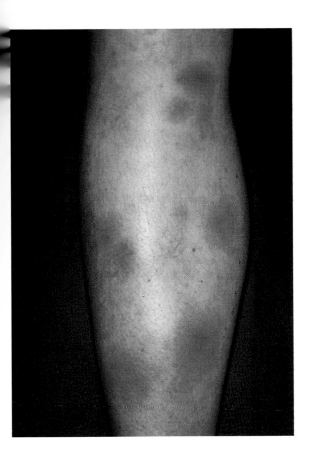

DRUG-INDUCED ERYTHEMA NODOSUM

Example chosen : **PARACETAMOL**

Painful deep-red subcutaneous nodules mainly on the anterior aspects of the legs (sometimes the forearms), typically in conjunction with fever and joint pains.
Other causes of erythema nodosum must also be considered (streptococcal infection, tuberculosis, sarcoidosis, Crohn's disease).

Drug-induced erythema nodosum: main drugs responsible

- Acetylsalicylic acid
- Iodides
- Oral contraceptives ?
- Paracetamol
- Sulfonamides

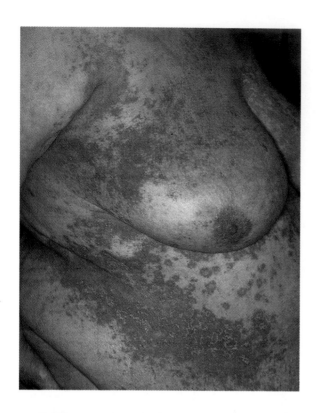

GENERALIZED PUSTULAR DERMATITIS

Example chosen: **DILTIAZEM**

A rash of multiple pustules on an erythematous background, beginning 1–2 days after initial exposure, on the face and flexure folds of the limbs, then spreading to involve the entire trunk.

After a few days (assuming drug withdrawal), the pustules dry and give way to extensive, and highly characteristic, superficial exfoliation, as after sunburn.

Histology shows intraepidermal pustules surrounded by spongiosis. Concomitant leukocytoclastic vasculitis is also often present.

A patch-test might be useful and often is positive. Reintroduction is not to be recommended.

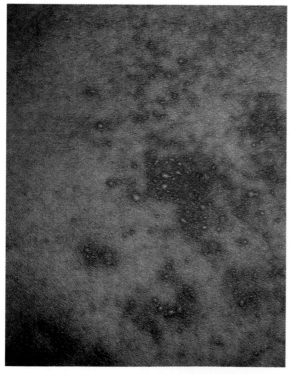

Generalized pustular dermatitis: main drugs responsible

- Antibiotics : Ampicillin, amoxicillin, cephalosporins, co-trimoxazole, doxycycline, imipenem, isoniazid
- Carbamazepine
- Diltiazem
- Furosemide
- Hydroxychloroquine

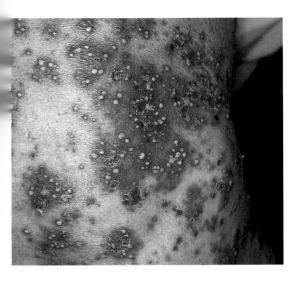

DRUG-INDUCED PUSTULAR OR PUSTULO-CRUSTY ERUPTION

A pustular eruption of sudden onset, usually after long-term treatment. In the case of bromides, the lesions commonly occur on the legs, leaving behind an extremely painful crusty hyperkeratosis which may make walking impossible.

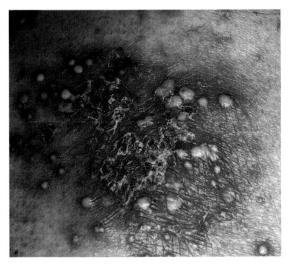

Pustular or pustulo-crusty eruption: main drugs responsible

- Halogens: Bromides, chlorides, halothane?
- Iodides

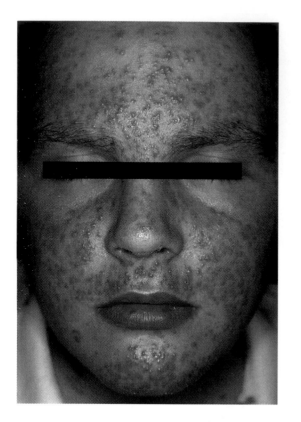

DRUG-INDUCED ACNEIFORM ERUPTION

Example chosen: **SYSTEMIC CORTICOSTEROIDS**

A papulo-pustular rash very similar to acne, and not confined to areas of high sebaceous gland density. Seborrhea and comedones are generally absent. The forehead and chin are usually involved. On the other hand, some drugs may exacerbate preexisting acne, in which case comedones will be present.

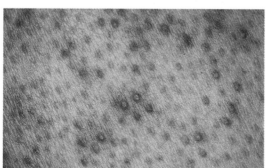

Acneiform rash: main drugs responsible
- ACTH
- Anabolic steroids
- Antitubercular agents: ethambutol, ethionamide
- Azathioprine
- Corticosteroids
- Lithium
- Vitamins B1 and B6 ?
- Vitamin B12

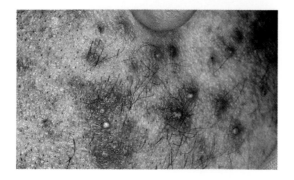

Preexisting acne: main drugs responsible
- Hydantoins
- Isoniazid
- Oral contraceptives
- Progestagens
- Testosterone

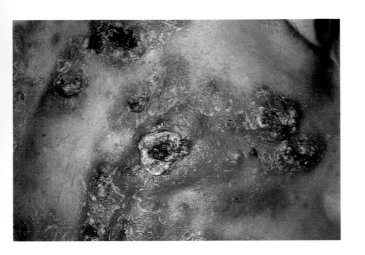

ISOTRETINOIN-INDUCED ACNE FULMINANS

Paradoxically and very rarely, isotretinoin may cause true acne fulminans (with fever, malaise and arthralgia).

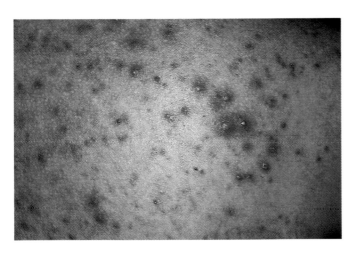

TETRACYCLINE-INDUCED GRAM-NEGATIVE FOLLICULITIS

Example chosen:
DOXYCYCLINE

Sudden onset of small follicular pustules on the back in an acne patient receiving long-term doxycycline. Pustules can also be seen at the base of the nose.

A swab from the pustules showed multiple Gram-negative organisms. An identical clinical picture may be caused by pityrosporal folliculitis (also commoner on long-term tetracycline therapy).

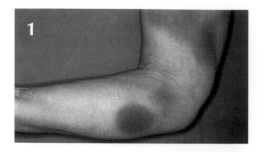

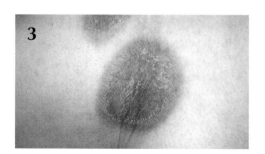

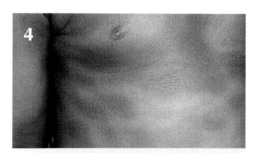

FIXED DRUG ERUPTION

Examples chosen:
ACETYLSALICYLIC ACID (Photos 1 to 4)
CO-TRIMOXAZOLE (Photo 5)

A sharply marginated, round or oval, erythematous or erythemato-purplish lesion recurring at the same site (Photo 1) a few hours to 1–2 days after exposure. The pigmentation deepens after several episodes (Photos 2 & 3). Pruritus or a burning sensation is present. The lesion is often single initially but other sites may subsequently become involved, even the entire skin surface (in particular in Blacks: Photo 4).

A fixed drug eruption may become bullous with subsequent erosion (in particular on mucous membranes). The penis is a highly characteristic site for this eventuality (Photo 5). Patch testing at the site can be considered. Reintroduction is entirely legitimate.

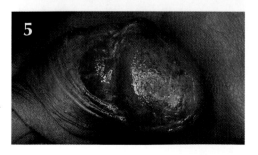

Fixed drug eruption: main drugs responsible

- Acetylsalicylic acid
- Amoxicillin
- Ampicillin
- Barbiturates
- Chlordiazepoxide
- Codeine
- Co-trimoxazole
- Dextromethorphan
- Hydantoin
- Hydralazine
- Metronidazole
- Nonsteroidal antiinflammatory drugs
- Paracetamol
- Phenolphthalein
- Tetracycline

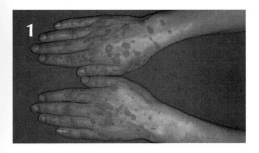

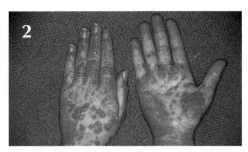

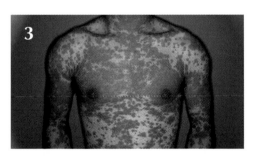

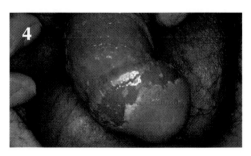

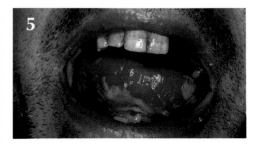

ERYTHEMA MULTIFORME AND STEVENS-JOHNSON SYNDROME

Example chosen: **CO-TRIMOXAZOLE**

These two entities are traditionally considered together on nosological grounds.

The papular lesions are usually round, distinct and symmetrical. Some have a variably prominent central bulla.

Usually drug-induced erythema multiforme is less typical than that which complicates viral infection (e.g. herpes). The hands (Photo 1), forearms and feet are usually involved (especially early in the eruption). Severe palmar erythema is highly characteristic (Photo 2). The entire skin surface may subsequently become invaded. Purpura may be present in addition to the bullae (Photo 3).

Stevens-Johnson syndrome is a severe bullous multi-orifice variant of erythema multiforme. Rapidly ulcerating bullae appear in the mouth, lips and genital mucous membranes, and sometimes on the ocular and nasal membranes. Fever, myalgia and arthralgia are also present. Hepatic enzyme levels may be abnormal (Photos 4 & 5).

Reintroduction is absolutely contra-indicated. Patch tests are usually negative or uninterpretable.

Erythema multiforme or Stevens-Johnson syndrome: main drugs responsible

- Barbiturates
- Carbamazepine
- Cephalosporins
- Co-trimoxazole
- Diltiazem
- Furosemide
- Hydantoins
- Nonsteroidal antiinflammatory drugs
- Pyrazoles
- Sulfones
- Thiazides

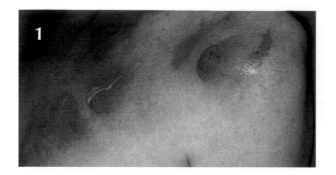

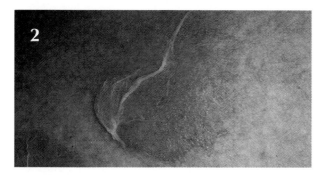

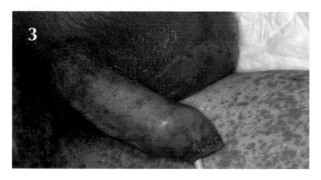

TOXIC EPIDERMAL NECROLYSIS (LYELL'S DISEASE)

Example chosen:
CARBAMAZEPINE

The dermis is rapidly bared by extensive exfoliation of fragile flaccid bullae (Photos 1 & 2). Prodromal symptoms (fever, cough, rhinitis, conjunctivitis and general malaise) are often present a few days before exfoliation begins. The condition usually begins with severe papular erythema or erythema multiforme (Photo 3), followed by the characteristic exfoliation. Nikolsky's sign (increase in bulla size in response to simple digital pressure or even on areas subject to friction) is positive. All skin areas except the scalp may be affected. The mucous membranes generally show major involvement (and may even be the site of the first lesions). Patients rapidly deteriorate, with major electrolyte loss. The prognosis must always be guarded. Transfer to a Burns Unit is mandatory given the frequency and severity of complications (in particular, sepsis). Onset is usually 1–3 weeks after drug exposure. Reintroduction is absolutely contraindicated although it has been reported that the reaction does not necessarily recur on accidental retreatment with the offending drug.

Toxic epidermal necrolysis: main drugs responsible

- Allopurinol
- Amoxicillin
- Ampicillin
- Barbiturates
- Carbamazepine
- Chlorpromazine
- Hydantoins
- Nitrofurantoin
- Nonsteroidal antiinflammatory drugs (especially oxicams)
- Sulfonamides (co-trimoxazole)

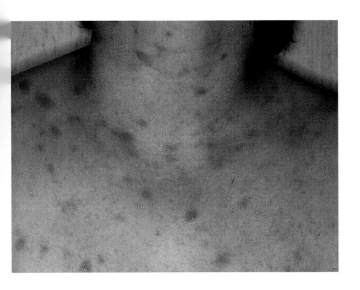

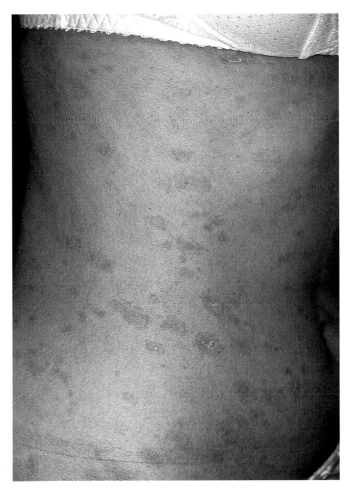

PITYRIASIS ROSEA-LIKE DRUG ERUPTION

Example chosen:

HYDROXYCHLOROQUINE

Multiple, roughly oval, erythemato-squamous patches distributed symmetrically over the body (mainly on the trunk). Trunk lesions have a marginal collarette of scale and a long axis running supero-inferiorly and postero-medially (i.e. parallel with the ribs).

If the offending drug is not withdrawn, the eruption may continue indefinitely and become refractory to all local treatment (in particular, corticosteroids). Unlike in the standard descriptions of Gibert's pityriasis rosea, there is no herald patch.

The interval between first exposure and onset can be several months.

Reintroduction may be attempted, and is in fact recommended to support the diagnosis.

Pityriasis rosea-like drug eruption: main drugs responsible

- Barbiturates
- Beta-blockers
- Bismuth
- Captopril
- Clonidine
- Gold salts
- Griseofulvin
- Ketotifen
- Metronidazole

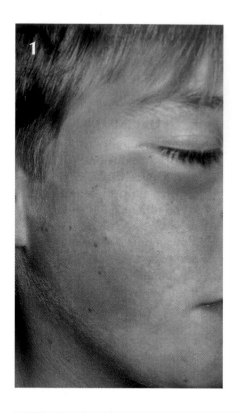

DRUG-INDUCED LUPUS ERYTHEMATOSUS

Example chosen: **CARBAMAZEPINE**

Scaly erythematous patches on the cheeks simulating authentic acute lupus erythematosus (Photo 1).

Cutaneous signs are only present in a small proportion of cases. There is marked photosensitivity and the areas most frequently involved are the face, upper arms and dorsa of the fingers (Photo 2). There may be concomitant Raynaud's syndrome.

Antinuclear factor and antihistone auto-antibodies are usually positive.

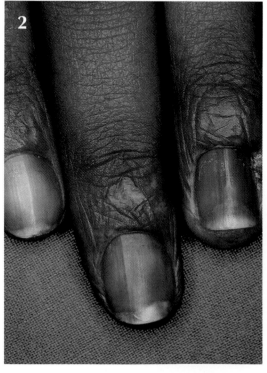

Drug-induced lupus erythematosus: main drugs responsible
- Beta-blockers
- Carbamazepine
- Hydantoins
- Hydralazine
- Isoniazid
- Methyldopa
- Minocyclin
- Penicillamine
- Procainamide
- Propylthiouracil

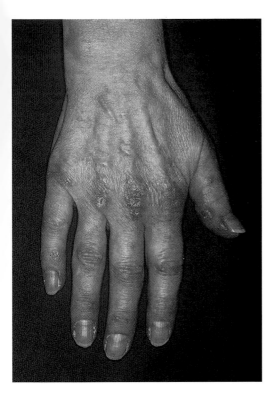

DRUG-INDUCED DERMATOMYOSITIS

Example chosen: **HYDROXYUREA**

Lesions identical to authentic dermatomyositis: periorbital purplish red heliotrope erythema and violaceous papules on the dorsa of the hands (knuckles, in particular) associated with periungual megacapillaries.

Drug-induced dermatomyositis: main drugs responsible
- BCG - Carbamazepine - Hydroxurea - Nonsteroidal antiinflammatory drugs - Penicillamine

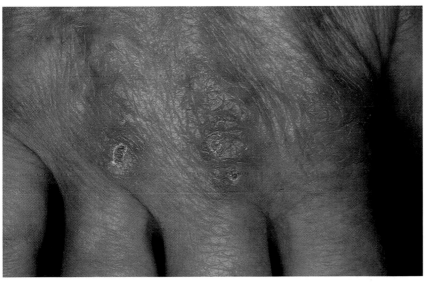

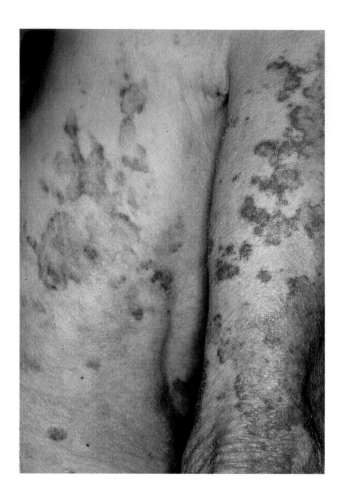

DRUG-INDUCED PEMPHIGUS

Example chosen:
PENICILLAMINE

Lesions identical to authentic pemphigus (clinical features, histology, immunofluorescence): large, flaccid, rapidly ulcerating bullae, some of which arise from apparently harmless erythematous or erythemato-crusty macules. The mouth is involved in over 50 % of cases.

Circulating auto-antibodies are found in the great majority of cases but are not essential to the diagnosis.

Drug-induced pemphigus generally, but not always, regresses slowly after withdrawal of the offending drug. Onset can be considerably delayed, occuring from 1 month to 5 years after initial exposure.

Drugs containing a thiol group tend to be most responsible.

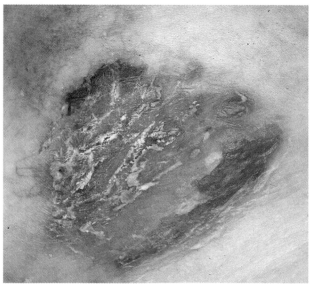

Drug-induced pemphigus: main drugs responsible

- Captopril
- Cephalosporins
- Gold salts
- Nifedipine
- Penicillamine
- Penicillins
- Piroxicam
- Pyritinol

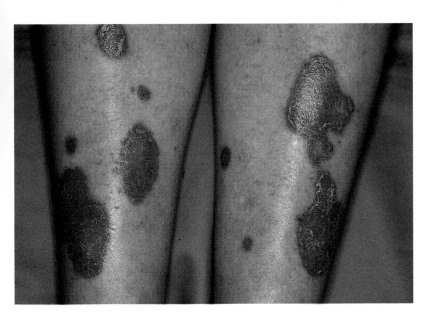

DRUG-INDUCED PSORIASIS

Example chosen: **LITHIUM**

Typical psoriasis-like eruption presenting as large, symmetrical, clearly marginated erythemato-squamous plaques months after initial exposure.

Whereas lithium appears able to trigger authentic psoriasis *de novo*, other drugs (see table) are most likely to trigger or exacerbate psoriasis in those already affected, possibly only 3–6 months after initial exposure. There is no reason not to attempt reintroduction.

Drug-induced psoriasis: main drugs responsible
- Angiotensin converting enzyme inhibitors
- Antimalarials
- Beta-blockers
- Chlorthalidone
- Clonidine
- Interferons
- Lithium
- Methyldopa
- Nonsteroidal antiinflammatory drugs

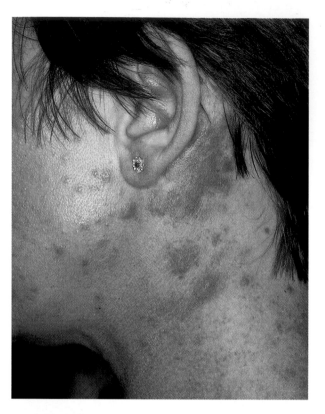

DRUG-INDUCED SWEET'S SYNDROME (ACUTE FEBRILE NEUTROPHILIC DERMATOSIS)

Example chosen: **MINOCYCLINE**

Pseudobullous erythemato-papular lesions with the formation of a fairly substantial superficial edema resembling incipient bullae. There is systemic involvement, with fever and myalgia. The sedimentation rate and neutrophil count are raised. Sweet's syndrome generally only occurs after prolonged treatment with the offending drug.

Sweet's syndrome: main drugs responsible
- GMCSF - Hydralazine - Minocycline

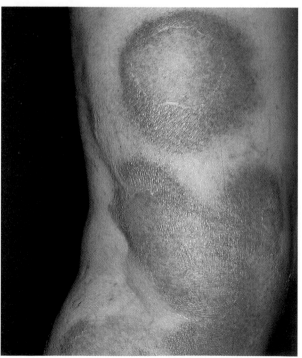

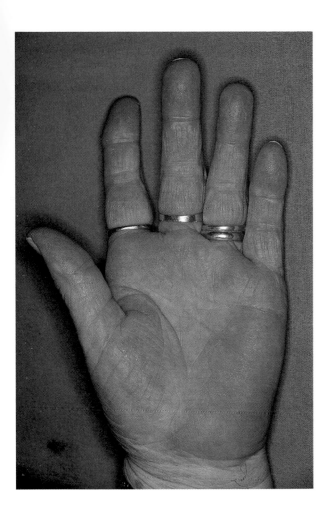

ANTIMITOTIC-INDUCED PALMAR (ACRAL) ERYTHEMA

Example chosen: **DOXORUBICIN**

Intense palmar (and sometimes plantar) erythema 1–2 days after dosing (Photo 1), particularly with rapid or bolus infusions of antimitotics. The erythema is dose-dependent. Bullae may occur. Reintroduction can be attempted. The reaction may be exacerbated by concomitant cyclosporin therapy. Other causes of palmar erythema must be searched for: pregnancy, liver disease, and active rheumatoid arthritis. It may also occur as an autosomal dominant disorder, or simply be idiopathic.

Palmar erythema: main drugs responsible

- Cyclosphosphamide
- Cytosine arabinoside
- Doxorubicin
- 5-fluorouracil
- Hydroxyurea
- Interleukin 2
- 6 Mercaptopurine
- Methotrexate

131

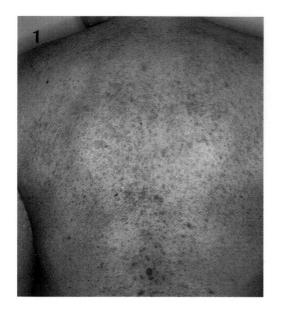

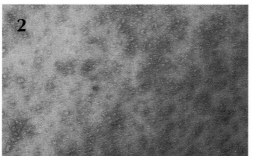

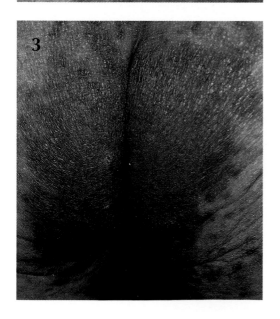

DRUG-INDUCED LICHENOID ERUPTION

Example chosen: **BETA-BLOCKER**

A generalized eruption of violaceous flat papules which may be topped by a network of whitish lines (Wickham's striae) resembling (idiopathic) lichen planus (Photos 1 & 2).

At points, the lesions often resemble eczema or psoriasis. In other cases (especially if the eruption has lasted a long time), the papules become distinctly confluent, brownish and purplish. In such cases, the lesions resemble poikiloderma (Photo 3). Pruritus is sometimes marked, but may be absent. Histology may be useful but again, the differential diagnosis with authentic idiopathic lichen planus may be difficult.

In most cases, onset occurs several months after initial exposure to the offending drug. Reintroduction may be attempted.

Lichenoid eruption: main drugs responsible

- Acyclovir
- Antimalarials
- Beta-blockers
- Captopril
- Furosemide
- Gold salts
- Isoniazid
- Methyldopa
- Piroxicam
- Quinidine
- Thiazides

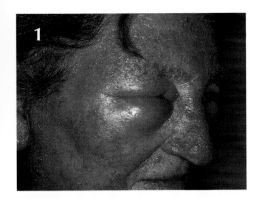

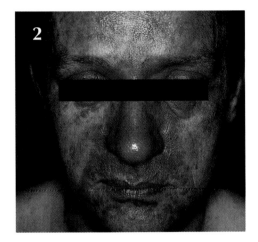

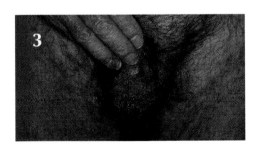

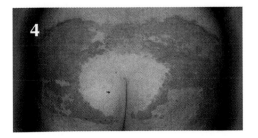

SYSTEMIC CONTACT DERMATITIS

A typically eczematous (papulo-vesicular exudative) generalized eruption 2–3 days after oral sulfonamide ingestion in a person previously sensitized transepidermally to another sulfonamide (cross-allergy).

The eyelids are often edematous (Photo 1). The sites previously involved (at the time of contact sensitization) are typically those where the reexacerbation occurs.

This type of generalized eruption may also occur after inhaling the substance responsible (example budesonide), in which case it begins mainly around the nose before becoming generalized (Photo 2). The same mechanism is seen in response to intravesical instillation of mitomycin : the eruption begins at the genital organs and medial aspects of the thighs before becoming generalized (Photo 3).

An improper term, "baboon syndrome", has often been used to denote a reaction of this type confined to the gluteal region and upper thigh and, on occasion, to the axilla.

Injectable antibiotics are usually responsible. These cases also depend on previous transepidermal sensitization : e.g. gentamycin injection in a patient presensitized to neomycin (Photo 4).

Systemic contact dermatitis: main drugs responsible

- Acyclovir
- Aminophylline
- Aminoglycosides
- Beta-blockers
- Budesonide
- Disulfiram
- Penicillins
- Phenothiazines
- Sulfonamide antibacterials
- Sulfonamide diuretics
- Sulfonylureas

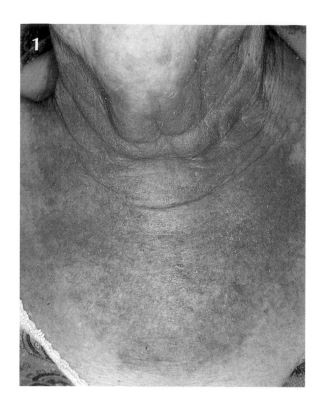

DRUG-INDUCED PHOTOSENSITIZATION ERUPTION

Clearly marginated papular erythema confined to exposed areas (upper chest, in this case) and resembling simple sunburn. There are no lesions on areas covered by clothes (Photo 1). This is an instance of dose-dependent phototoxic erythema ("dose", in this case, referring to both drug and sunlight). The erythema can be severe and take on a distinctly purple hue (Photo 2). There may be an associated 'flu-like illness. Bullous exfoliation may occur. Phototoxic accidents are common in the fingernails given their absence of melanin, and present as distal detachment (photo-onycholysis, Photo 3). Phototoxic eruptions occur within hours of irradiation.

Much less often, authentic photo-allergic reactions mimick contact dermatitis in sunlight-exposed areas. The lesion margins are less distinct in such cases; there is considerable pruritus. Lesion onset is 2–3 days after exposure to sunlight (Photos 4 & 5).

Photopatch tests are positive in all cases.

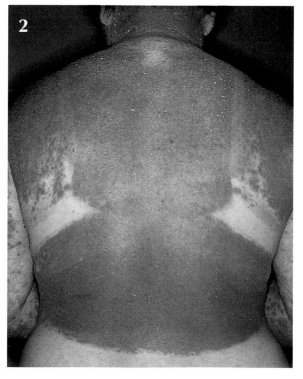

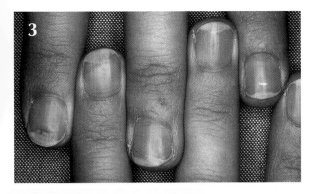

In practice most photosensitization accidents are phototoxic in origin while all drugs causing photo-allergy can also be phototoxic. Reintroduction must not be attempted on any account as it could be followed by residual photosensitization.

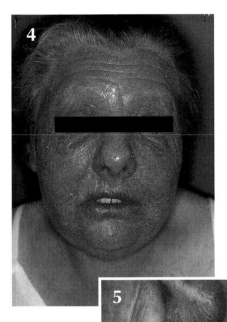

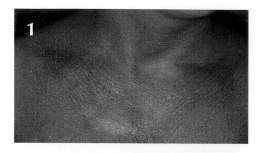

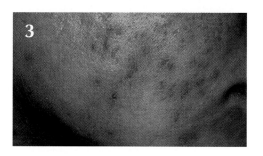

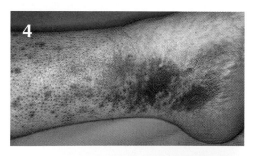

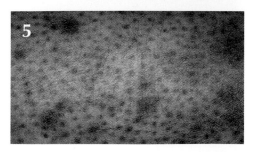

DRUG-INDUCED HYPERPIGMENTATION

ACTH (Photos 1 & 2)

Brownish, variably reticular, "dirty" pigmentation, mainly of the neck ("dirty neck"), and reminiscent of Addison's disease. This highly specific type of pigmentation is due to high-dose ACTH injection. The palmar folds may also be affected. The pigmentation is essentially melanocytic.

MINOCYCLINE (Photos 3 to 6)

Blueish pigmentation of old acne scars, resulting from long-term minocycline therapy (Photo 3).
This type of blackish-blue minocycline pigmentation may also occur on lower limbs (Photos 4 & 5), or on mucous membranes, in which case the pigmentation is brownish (Photo 6). These various types of hyperpigmentation disappear slowly after treatment withdrawal.

ANTIMALARIALS (Photos 7 & 8)

Bluish, slate-blue or brownish pigmentation induced by synthetic antimalarials. This highly distinctive pigmentation is only observed after treatment for several months, generally at high doses (Photo 7). The nails may sometimes be involved, exhibiting wide bluish bands (Photo 8).
Identical pigmentation may be found on the palate.

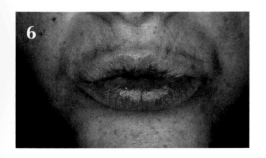

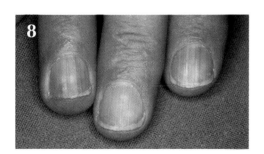

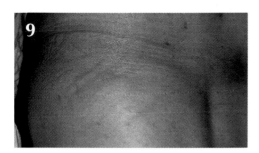

BLEOMYCIN (Photo 9)

Flagellate brownish pigmentation induced by bleomycin: high doses are often necessary. The reaction disappears slowly after drug withdrawal.

SILVER SALTS (Photo 10)

Slate-gray pigmentation due to long-term silver salt ingestion (argyria), clearly visible on the mucous membranes (especially the mouth) and nails.

Hyperpigmentation: main drugs responsible

- ACTH
- Amiodarone
- Antimalarials
- Bismuth
- Chlorpromazine
- Clofazimine
- Cytostatics
- Hydantoins
- Methyldopa
- Minocyclin
- Oral contraceptives
- Silver salts

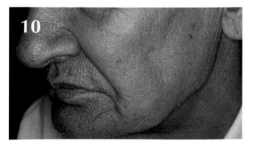

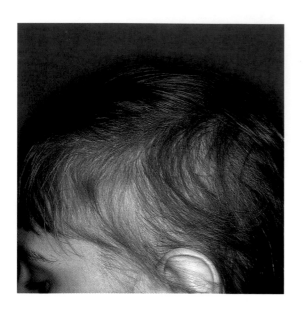

DRUG-INDUCED DIFFUSE ALOPECIA

Example chosen: **BETA-BLOCKER**

Diffuse alopecia, beginning at the vertex and gradually spreading to the entire scalp. Most drugs cause alopecia by telogen effluvium, a term used to describe the shedding of normal club hairs following the premature precipitation of anagen follicles into telogen (a common follicle response to many types of stress). Cytostatics differ in giving rise to both an anagen and telogen effluvium. In the latter case, alopecia onset occurs soon after dosing whereas with the other drugs it occurs only after a long interval (often several months).

Diffuse alopecia: main drugs responsible
- Allopurinol
- Amitriptyline
- Amphetamines and derivatives
- Beta-blockers
- Carbamazepine
- Carbimazole
- Cimetidine
- Colchicine
- Coumarins
- Cytostatics
- Doxepine
- Fibrates (especially clofibrate)
- Fluoxetine
- Flupentixol
- Heparin
- Hydantoins
- Isotretinoin
- Levodopa
- Nonsteroidal antiinflammatory drugs
- Oral contraceptives ?
- Propylthiouracil
- Valproate

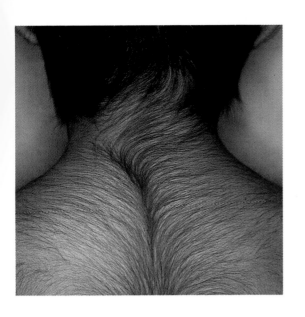

DRUG-INDUCED HYPERTRICHOSIS

Example chosen: **CYCLOSPORIN**

Cyclosporin-induced hypertrichosis after some 6 months therapy (Photo 1).
Hair growth reverses slowly after drug withdrawal.
In contrast to hirsutism, hypertrichosis is not due to an increase in androgen production. Reversibility of drug-induced hirsutism is much more unpredictable.

Hypertrichosis: main drugs responsible

- Cyclosporin
- Diazoxide (especially in children)
- Minoxidil (both topical and systemic administration)
- Penicillamine
- Psoralens

Hirsutism: main drugs responsible

- ACTH
- Androgens
- Corticosteroids
- Hydantoins
- Progestagens

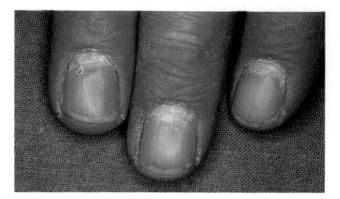

Onychomadesis (shedding) of the proximal part of the nail.

RETINOID-INDUCED NAIL LESIONS

Retinoids (especially acitretin) can cause many acquired nail lesions which always reverse after treatment withdrawal.

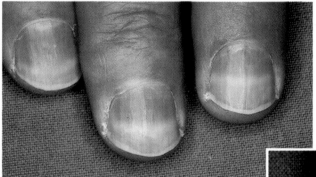

Transverse leukonychia.

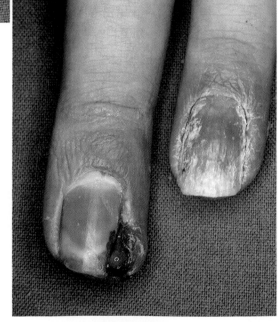

Periungual pyogenic granuloma in a psoriasis patient receiving acitretin.

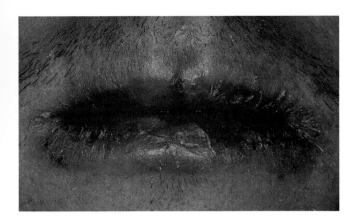

RETINOID-INDUCED CHEILITIS

Dry sparsely fissured cheilitis occurs in virtually all patients on retinoid therapy and is dose-dependent. It is due to a direct effect of retinoids on the sebaceous glands and is mainly observed with isotretinoin.

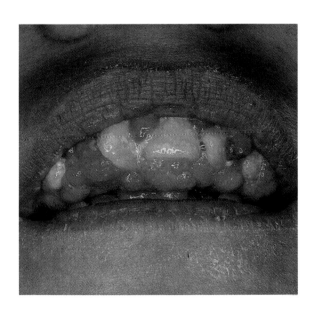

DRUG-INDUCED GINGIVAL HYPERPLASIA

Example chosen: **CYCLOSPORIN**

Drug-induced gingival hyperplasia generally begins only after treatment has been taken for 3–6 months. It may be substantial, and a cause of some inconvenience. It presents initially as interdental papillae: the patient complains of pain and bleeding on the slightest friction, e.g. when brushing the teeth. In principle it is dose-dependent and regresses slowly on treatment withdrawal.

Gingival hyperplasia: main drugs responsible

- Cyclosporin
- Diltiazem
- Hydantoins
- Nifedipine

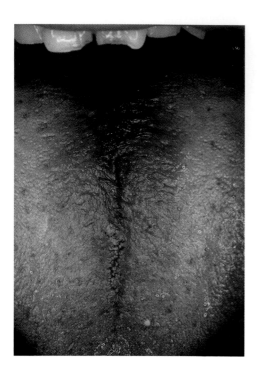

DRUG-INDUCED BLACK HAIRY TONGUE

Example chosen: **SPIRAMYCIN**

Photo 1. Brown to blackish coloration associated with hyperplasia and hyperkeratosis of the filiform papillae of the tongue. The condition may be idiopathic, but is also observed weeks after treatment with certain drugs, mainly antibiotics.
Colonization by *Candida albicans* is only secondary.

Black hairy tongue: main drugs responsible

- Antibiotics (various, but especially broad spectrum)
- Griseofulvin

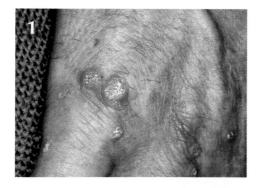

ARSENIC-INDUCED SIMPLE AND BOWENOID KERATOSIS

Keratotic lesions on the dorsa of the hands 2–3 years after taking large amounts of potassium arsenite (Fowler's solution) for psoriasis (Photo 1). The lesions can degenerate to squamous cell carcinoma.
Bowenoid keratosis (Photo 2) developing more than 10 years after long-term arsenical therapy: multiple, rounded and slightly infiltrated lesions spreading slowly in various areas of the skin. Untreated lesions progress to squamous cell carcinoma.

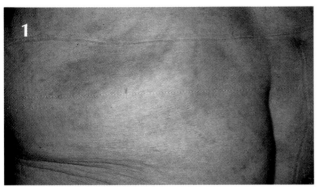

CUTANEOUS HEMOSIDEROSIS

Locally, iron injections can cause an authentic brownish tattoo (hemosiderosis) which is generally irreversible (Photos 1 & 2). Pigmentation induced by injections of sclerosants (polidocanol) to treat varicose veins (Photos 3 & 4). It is due mainly to hemosiderin, and reverses very slowly and sometimes only partially.

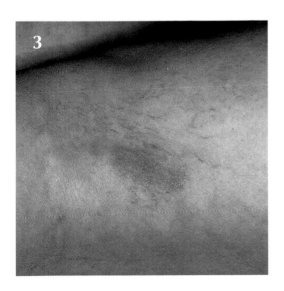

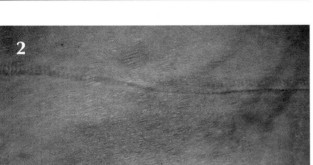

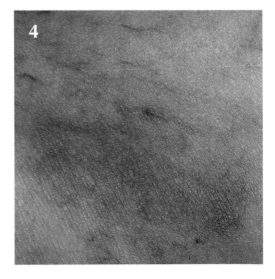

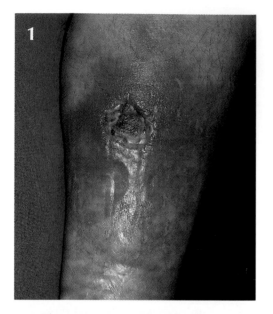

CUTANEOUS ULCERATION DUE TO PARAVENOUS INJECTION

Examples chosen:
POLIDOCANOL (photo 1) and DOXORUBICIN (photos 2 to 4)

Photo 1.
Large necrotic ulcer surrounded by extensive inflammatory erythema after paravenous injection of an excess concentration of polidocanol.

Photo 2.
Large blisters surrounded by intense inflammation resembling chemical cellulitis caused by extravasation of doxorubicin, with associated severe pain and loss of function.

Photo 3.
As above, a few days later: large ulcers with a fibrinous base, and severe persistent pain. Referral for plastic surgery is mandatory.

Photo 4.
Massive necrosis in the breast 2 weeks after para-jugular injection of doxorubicin. Mastectomy was required.

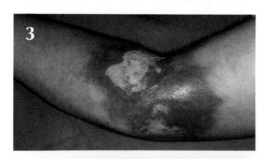

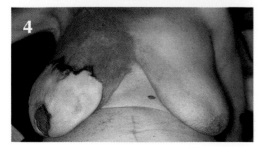

Cutaneous ulceration due to paravenous injection: main drugs responsible

- Bleomycin
- Cisplatin
- Dacarbazine
- Doxorubicin
- 5-fluorouracil
- Methotrexate

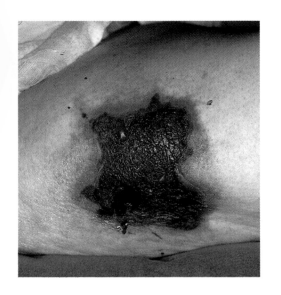

CUTANEOUS ULCERATION DUE TO ACCIDENTAL INTRA-ARTERIAL INJECTION

Example chosen: **NONSTEROIDAL ANTIINFLAMMATORY DRUG**

Aseptic necrosis 10 days after accidental intra-arterial injection of an NSAID. At the time of the injection the patient felt violent pain. The initial appearance was that of intense well-demarcated erythema reminiscent of localized livedo (Nicolau's livedoid dermatitis). Necrosis and ulceration only occurred later.

Cutaneous ulceration due to accidental intra-arterial injection: main drugs responsible

- Chlorpromazine
- Corticosteroids
- Nonsteroidal antiinflammatory drugs

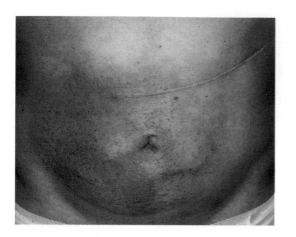

NICKEL CONTACT DERMATITIS DUE TO SUBCUTANEOUS DESFERRIOXAMINE INFUSION

Exudative erythemato-vesicular dermatitis due to nickel in the desferrioxamine solution (used to treat thalassemia major). The patient was presensitized to nickel. The nickel sulfate patch test was positive.

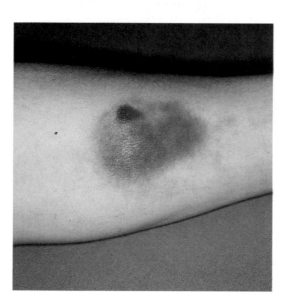

COLD ABSCESS AND GRANULOMA FOLLOWING BCG INJECTION

Large, slightly resistant mass developing 4–6 weeks after BCG therapy. Intradermal BCG may sometimes cause a cold abscess which is very slow to resorb. Lymphadenopathy is also present and may be painful. This type of complication is mainly seen in patients strongly sensitized to tuberculin or in those who receive amounts which are excessive and/or injected too deep.

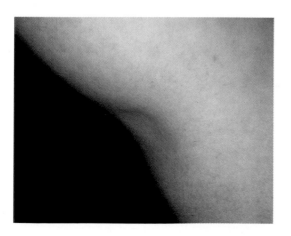

LIPODYSTROPHY DUE TO INSULIN INJECTION

Deep atrophy (lipoatrophy) due to repeated depot insulin injection at the same site. The lesion is irreversible once it has reached this stage.

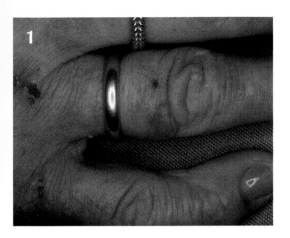

PSEUDO PORPHYRIA CUTANEA TARDA AND HEMODIALYSIS

Bullous dermatosis mimicking the clinical and histological features of authentic porphyria cutanea tarda. The bullae form on light-exposed areas (face, neckline and dorsa of hands), which soon become extremely painful. There may be associated milia (Photos 1 & 2). The condition occurs after several months of hemodialysis and may be associated with elevation of blood and urinary porphyrins.

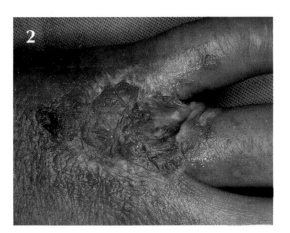

The adverse cutaneous effects of PUVA therapy may be acute or chronic. Acute effects are essentially burns due to overdosage (of either psoralen or UVA).

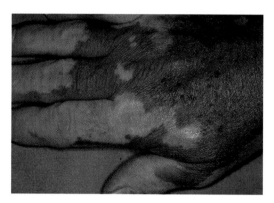

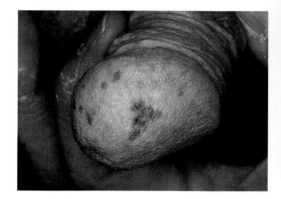

Erythema of depigmented areas (vitiligo) and grossly accentuated pigmentation of non depigmented areas (normal skin) due to an excessive number of PUVA sessions in a nonresponder treated for vitiligo.

PUVA-induced lentigines of the glans penis caused by an excessive total dose. The genitalia should always be protected from UVA to prevent this complication. Squamous cell carcinoma may also develop.

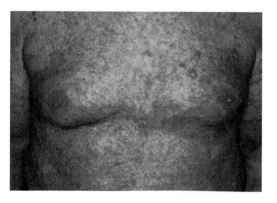

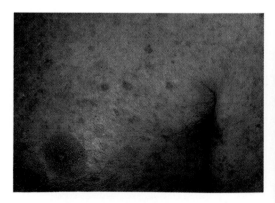

Pigmented xerodermoid (dry skin and multiple lentigines) in a psoriatic patient who had undergone many PUVA sessions, to a total dose of over 4000 Joules/cm2.

LOCAL AND GENERAL SIDE EFFECTS OF TOPICAL CORTICOSTEROIDS

The intensive use of corticosteroids in dermatological therapy justifies a section on their local side effects. In the vast majority of cases, the effects are due either to fairly long-term use of a potent steroid or by repeated application to an area particularly prone to side effects (face, major skin folds, genital organs etc).

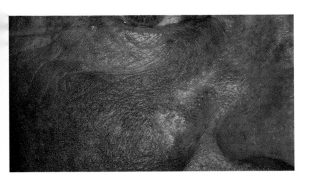

STEROID RUBEOSIS

Papular erythema and multiple telangiectases on the face after applying a potent corticosteroid for several weeks. Some atrophic areas are also present: the skin is hypersensitive with a sensation of nagging pain and burning.

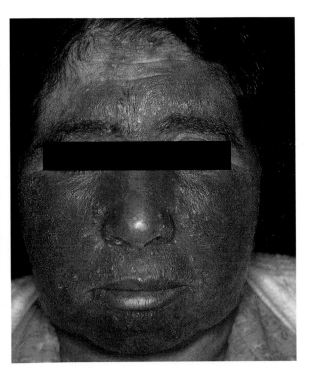

STEROID ROSACEA

Pan-facial papulo-pustular erythema due to potent steroid application for several months. The condition is both steroid-induced and steroid-dependent: at each attempt at steroid withdrawal, the rosacea worsens markedly. Oral therapy is essential (tetracycline, metronidazole or isotretinoin).

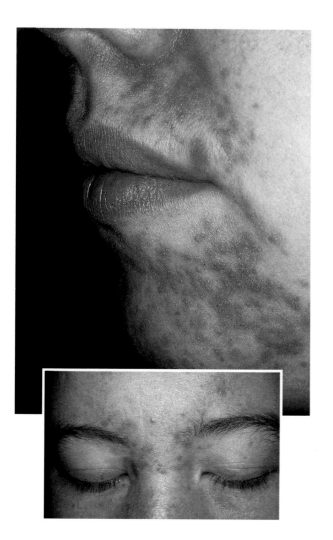

STEROID PERIORAL DERMATITIS

Multiple distinct papulo-pustules around the mouth leaving a narrow unaffected area near the semi-mucous membranes of the lips. Erythema is intense. The paranasal furrows are often involved.
Perioral dermatitis is a classic side effect of topical steroid therapy for seborrheic dermatitis of the ala nasi, often with onset after treatment for only a few days or weeks. In some cases, the glabellar area is involved.

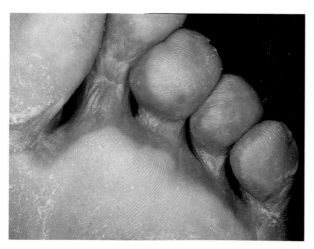

STEROID ATROPHY

Glazed erythema on a background of an atrophic plantar interdigital web. The whitish desquamation in the cleft is due to dermatophytosis. Burning sensations and pruritus are also present. This type of atrophy is seen only after long periods of potent corticosteroid use. It reverses slowly.

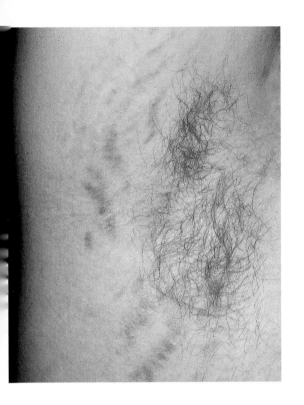

STEROID STRIAE

Erythema and linear atrophy caused by fairly prolonged use of a potent corticosteroid in a major skin fold (in this case the axilla).

On steroid withdrawal, the erythematous component reverses slowly, giving way to permanent whitish atrophy.

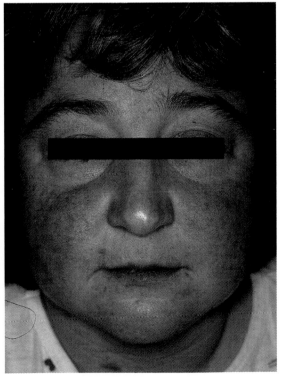

CUSHING'S SYNDROME DUE TO TOPICAL CORTICOSTEROIDS

In rare cases, intensive application of (even weak) local corticosteroids may trigger authentic iatrogenic Cushing's syndrome. This complication is most frequently seen in young children in whom daily application of large amounts of corticosteroids to the entire skin surface can inhibit the hypothalamo-hypophyseal-adrenal axis followed, at a later stage, by authentic Cushing's syndrome with facial edema. In children, the syndrome is also associated with major height and weight retardation.

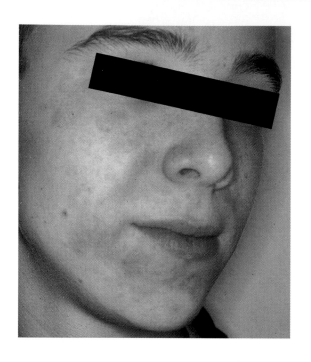

IRRITANT DERMATITIS: TOPICAL TRETINOIN

Dry diffuse facial erythema appearing soon after using local tretinoin to prevent and treat photoaging. Excess concentrations cause uncomfortable and photosensitive irritant dermatitis, with a local burning sensation. The dermatitis is strictly confined to the treated areas.

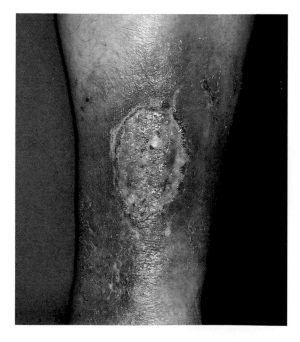

IRRITANT DERMATITIS: SWABS CONTAINING EXCESSIVE COPPER SULFATE

Intense peri-ulcer erythema appearing soon after prolonged use of wet swabs containing inadequately diluted copper sulfate (used as a detergent in the treatment of a leg ulcer).

ALLERGIC CONTACT DERMATITIS TO LOCAL ANTISEPTICS AND ANTIBIOTICS

Local antiseptics and antibiotics are often responsible for allergic contact dermatitis.

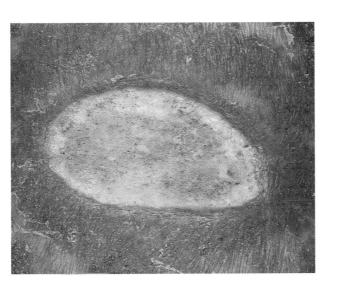

ALLERGIC CONTACT DERMATITIS: HEXAMIDINE

Multiple pruritic papular vesicles 3 days after a single application of hexamidine to disinfect a cauterization wound.
Hexamidine often causes follicular eczema. The hexamidine patch test was positive.

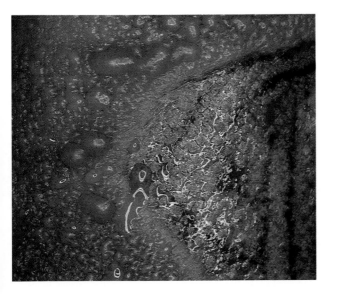

ALLERGIC CONTACT DERMATITIS: CHLORHEXIDINE

Characteristic allergic contact dermatitis to chlorhexidine after dermabrasion tattoo removal. Pruritus is intense. Dermabrasion probably contributed by facilitating allergen penetration.
The chlorhexidine patch test was positive.

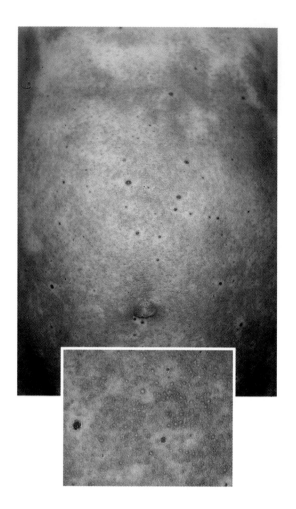

ALLERGIC CONTACT DERMATITIS: MERCURY

Extensive contact dermatitis a few days after using a solution containing a mercury antiseptic to dry varicella vesicles. Pruritus is intense (merging with the symptoms of varicella). Note the non involvement of the areas surrounding the varicella lesions (crusting in this photograph), probably due to the cutaneous vasculitic microinfarcts caused by the Herpes zoster virus infection. The ammoniated mercury patch test was positive.

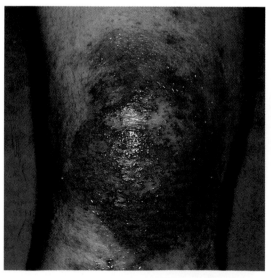

ALLERGIC CONTACT DERMATITIS: CHLORAMPHENICOL

Heavily exudative papulo-vesicular erythema 72 hours after using a 2 % chloramphenicol ointment to disinfect a traumatic knee wound. The chloramphenicol patch test was positive.

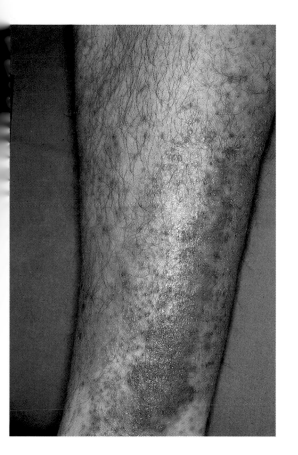

ALLERGIC CONTACT DERMATITIS: NEOMYCIN

Papulo-vesicular purpuric dermatitis of the leg after applying a neomycin cream. The neomycin patch test was positive.

ALLERGIC CONTACT DERMATITIS
DUE TO ANTIVIRALS

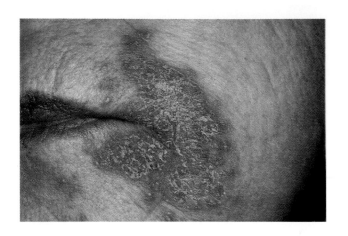

ALLERGIC CONTACT DERMATITIS: TROMANTADINE

Chronic pruritic dry erythema with distant lesions, caused by long-term tromantadine application as a local treatment for peribuccal herpes.
The tromantadine patch test was positive.

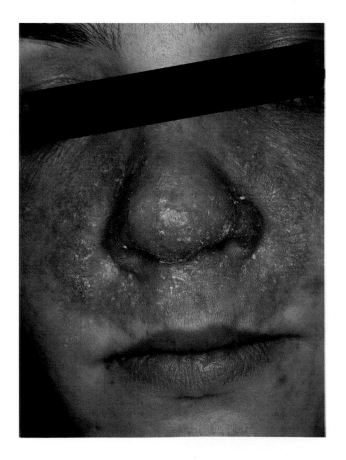

ALLERGIC CONTACT DERMATITIS: ACYCLOVIR CREAM

Extensive allergic contact dermatitis at the acute vesicular exudative stage involving the entire nose with some extension to the cheeks. In the present case, the contact dermatitis was not due to acyclovir itself but to the propylene glycol in the excipient (which aids the absorption of acyclovir). Patch tests were positive with the cream itself and propylene glycol, and negative with acyclovir.

ALLERGIC CONTACT DERMATITIS DUE TO TOPICAL ANTIINFLAMMATORIES AND RUBEFACIENTS

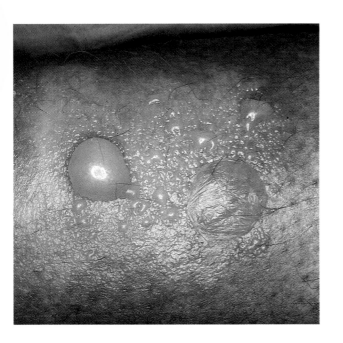

ALLERGIC CONTACT DERMATITIS: KETOPROFEN

Vesiculo-bullous plaque on an inflammatory background soon after topical ketoprofen therapy for a sprain in a young athlete (Photo 1). There was severe associated pruritus. The lesion was markedly exacerbated by light. The ketoprofen patch test was positive. The photopatch test (with UVA) confirmed exacerbation by light.

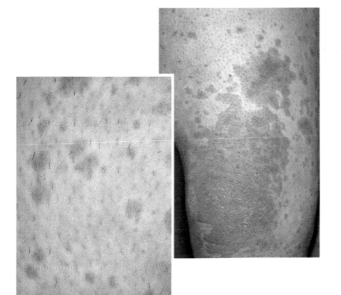

ALLERGIC CONTACT DERMATITIS: MEPHENESINE

Papular erythema with small peripheral lesions. All lesions are surrounded by a vasoconstriction halo reminiscent of pseudo erythema multiforme.
This particular type of contact allergy is often seen with mephenesine (used as a rubefacient for muscle pains in athletes).
The mephenesine patch test was positive.

ALLERGIC CONTACT DERMATITIS TO TRANSDERMAL THERAPEUTIC SYSTEMS (TTS)

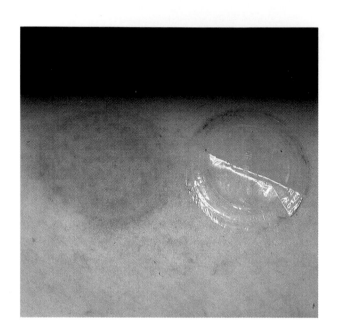

ALLERGIC CONTACT DERMATITIS: ESTROGEN TTS

Microvesicular erythema (and marked pruritus) consistently occurring 24–48 hours after applying an estrogen-containing TTS.
The dermatitis spreads beyond the confines of the TTS itself. Patch tests to the TTS and estrogen were positive. The alternative routes of administration are oral and paren-teral.

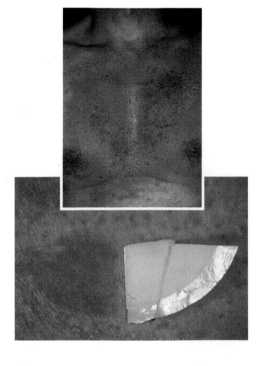

ALLERGIC CONTACT DERMATITIS: NICOTINE TTS

Major exudative erythemato-vesicular derma-titis extending over the entire anterior aspect of the trunk with some identical lesions on the limbs, after treatment for 1 month with a TTS containing nicotine (to aid tobacco with-drawal).
The patch test to the TTS itself was strongly positive. This is a case of nicotine allergy. The adhesive acrylic resins in the TTS may have been responsible. This is another instance of the vital contribution of patch tests in pin-pointing the allergen responsible.

ALLERGIC CONTACT DERMATITIS DUE TO OTHER TOPICAL DRUGS

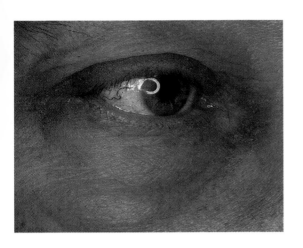

ALLERGIC CONTACT DERMATITIS: BETA-BLOCKER

Palpebral vesicular edema on an erythematous background. Associated allergic conjunctivitis is common. Pruritus is severe. Repeated use of a topical beta-blocker (against glaucoma) may cause contact sensitization. The beta-blocker patch test was positive. On the eyebrows, contact allergy often involves varying degrees of edema. Contact sensitization to the beta-blocker may develop after months of use, often delaying and complicating the diagnosis.

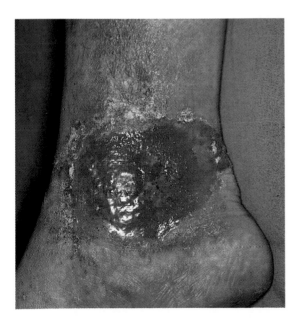

ALLERGIC CONTACT DERMATITIS: LANOLIN

Marked erythema with multiple exudative vesicles on the ankle due to sensitization to wool fat (lanolin) in a treatment for hyperkeratosis and dry skin.
The lanolin patch test was positive. Lanolin should no longer be used (especially to treat leg ulcers or stasis dermatitis), given its allergenic potential (Photo 4).

IX. DERMATOSES CAUSED BY INFECTIONS AND PARASITES

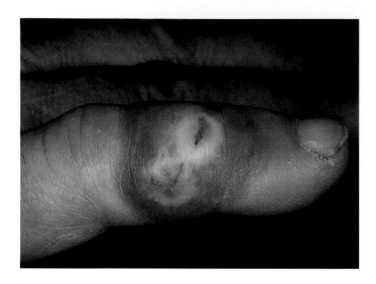

ORF

Orf is a disease of sheep and, more rarely, goats caused by a parapoxvirus. Transmission is well-documented to humans, in whom it is an occupational disease due to direct contact with either sick animals or contaminated objects.

Human disease presents as a slightly umbilicated purplish nodule 1–2 cm in diameter with a vesiculo-pustular roof.

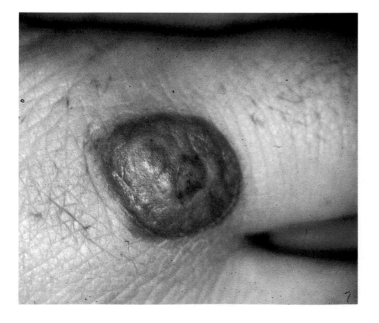

MILKER'S NODULE

The human variant of infection by the (orf-related) parapoxvirus responsible for pseudocowpox in cattle. Transmission occurs during milking. Clinically the lesions – large purplish nodules with a crust over the depressed centre – resemble orf.

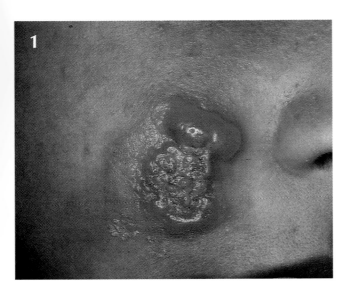

HERPES SIMPLEX AND ENVIRONMENT

Herpes simplex is caused by two types of *Herpes hominis* virus : type I, responsible for classic herpes, and type II, responsible for genital herpes, though the division between these two variants is not watertight, given the diversification of sexual practice in the population.
Herpes simplex is characterized by a primary infection, with potential recurrences (recurrent herpes). Environmental factors triggering both primary infection and recurrences include sunlight (and ultraviolet light), together with occupational hazards, in particular in health care workers exposed to herpes lesions.

Photo 1.
Recurrent vesiculo-bullous solar herpes on a thick erythematous base in a child. This was a second recurrence, at the start of a winter sports holiday.

Photo 2.
Recurrent herpes of the finger in a female nurse. Coalescent vesicles gradually transforming to pustules have developed on a very painful erythemato-edematous plaque.

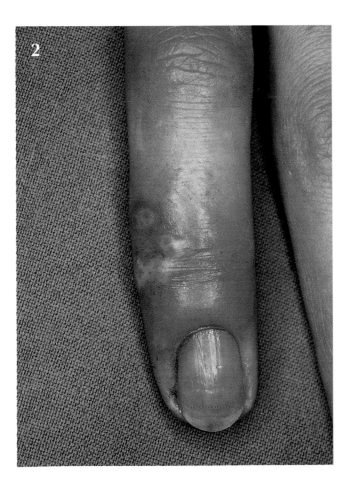

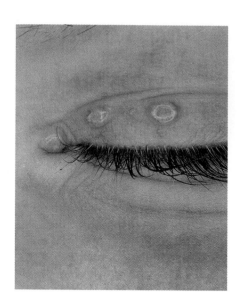

MOLLUSCUM CONTAGIOSUM

Molluscum contagiosum is caused by a poxvirus, three types of which have been identified to date. Infection is extremely common in childhood and presents as round, umbilicated, often shiny, smooth-surfaced papules a few millimeters in diameter. Initially they contain whitish creamy material which spontaneously discharges, after which the lesions crust over and are eventually destroyed.

They are extremely contagious and often multiple. They are particularly common in children with atopic dermatitis, as illustrated.

It has often been claimed, though remains to be proved, that increased use of swimming pools by children accounts for the current increase in frequency.

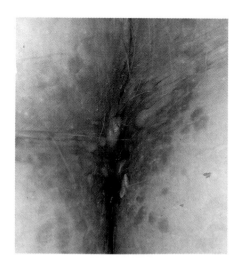

CONDYLOMATA ACUMINATA (ANOGENITAL WARTS)

Transmission is essentially sexual. The pathogen is human papillomavirus (HPV) 6 or 11. In children they may be the result of sexual abuse, but they can also occur spontaneously. They usually present as reddish fleshy masses, more rarely as multiple flesh-coloured sessile papular lesions (illustrated), developing as in this case on an erythematous base due to perianal maceration.

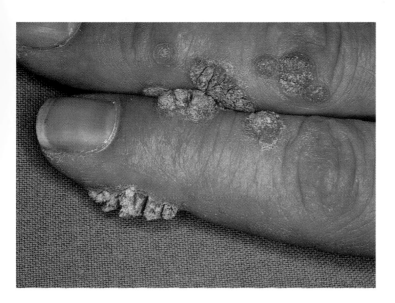

Warts on the lateral aspects of the fingers in a butcher, showing far advanced craggy keratosis.

BUTCHER'S WARTS

Hand warts are frequent and multiple in butchers and poultry carcase processors, in whom they constitute an authentic occupational disease due in most cases to HPV 7, though on occasion to other types. This is not a case of transmission of an animal papillomavirus to man, but of interhuman transmission, favoured by a combination of environmental factors including work in a humid environment, at relatively low temperature and with frequent microtrauma.

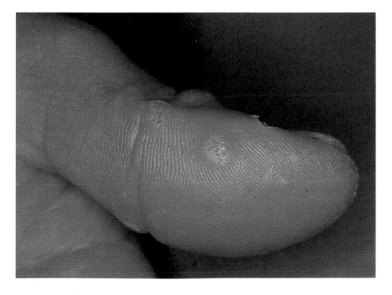

Warts on the palmar aspect of the fingers in a poultry processor. They resemble the myrmeciae of HPV 1 infection: endophytic lesions surrounded by a small ring of keratosis with central black dots representing thrombosed capillaries.

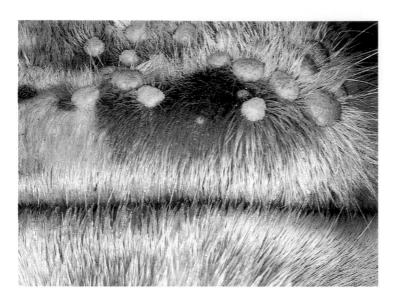

Viral papillomata around the lips in a horse: multiple non keratotic shiny-domed papules. In other cases they appear much more wart-like, and similar to those found in cattle.

ANIMAL PAPILLOMATA

Many animals (cattle, horses, dogs, rabbits, sheep, deer) can be carriers of possibly species-specific wart viruses. Transmission of an animal papillomavirus to man has never been proved.

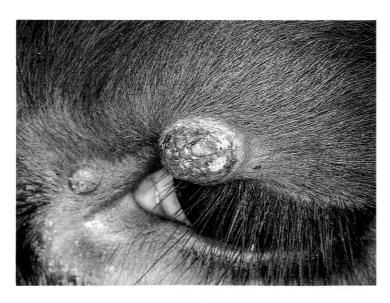

Viral papillomata in a cow. Highly keratotic round papules, similar in appearance to various common warts found in man. In some cases the warts may converge into plaques several centimeters in diameter.

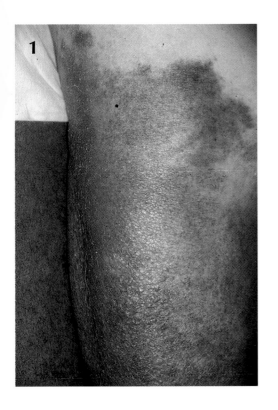

ERYSIPELAS OF THE LEG

The primary feature is the appearance of diffusely marginated erythematous edema (Photo 1) which is warm and painful and may be scattered with tense bullae (Photo 2). The eruption is sometimes associated with a high temperature and general malaise. Traditionally held to be streptococcal in origin, erysipelas is nowadays more often ascribed to mixed flora comprising both Gram +ve and -ve bacteria. The portal of entry in most cases is either a plantar inter-digital fissure (harbouring mixed flora: dermatophytes + bacteria) or trauma. Given this range of pathogens, erysipelas warrants broad spectrum antibiotic therapy.

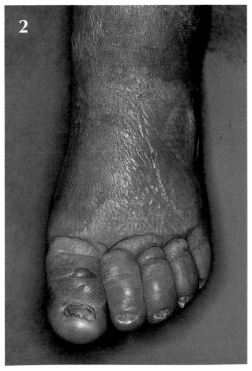

BACTERIAL ATHLETE'S FOOT

The commonest cause of this purely bacterial variant is a mixture of flora comprising both Gram +ve and -ve bacteria. The clinical presentation can be florid, with the entire inter-digital web and neighbouring skin subject to extensive ulceration with raised, whitish and macerated margins. It may be associated with small fissures in the clefts providing a portal of entry for erysipelas of the leg. Athlete's foot is a misnomer, as both water sports and occlusive (maceration-promoting) high-an-kled trainers also contribute to this environmental dermatosis.

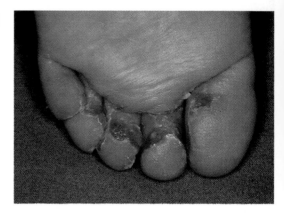

PSEUDOMONAS AERUGINOSA FOLLICULITIS

Epidemics of *P. aeruginosa* folliculitis are now commonly associated with aquatic activities, particularly public jacuzzis (pH > 8 and only 2–3 g free chlorine, which is inadequate at this pH) or inadequately chlorinated swimming pools. *P. aeruginosa* is an organism universally present in humid environments.

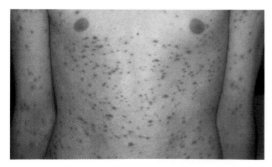

Papulo-pustular eruption of fulminant onset on the trunk of a teenage frequenter of public jacuzzis. As the lesions are perfectly symmetrical, the differential diagnosis is a drug eruption. The fact that the lesions all appeared simultaneously excludes a diagnosis of varicella.

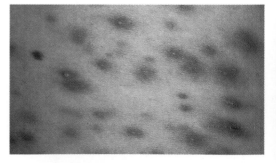

Close-up documenting a papulo-pustular eruption. The microbiology confirmed *P. aeruginosa* infection.

COSMOPOLITAN ATYPICAL MYCOBACTERIOSIS

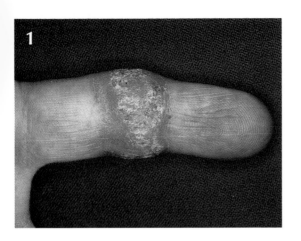

MYCOBACTERIUM MARINUM MYCOBACTERIOSIS: AQUARIUM GRANULOMA

A condition found almost exclusively in fish fanciers. The portal of entry is a minor wound which may go unnoticed. The lesion presents either as a bright-red single nodule which is mildly keratotic (Photo 1) or as coalescent purplish red plaques (Photo 2) of the fingers or dorsum of the hand. A fairly common clinical variant is the sporotrichoid form, in which one or several satellite nodules appear at succesive intervals on the forearm along the line of lymph drainage (Photo 3), sometimes in association with locoregional lymphadenopathy.

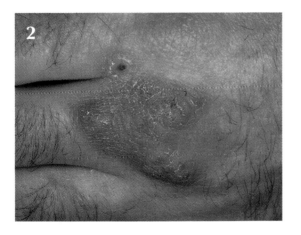

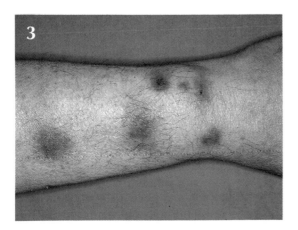

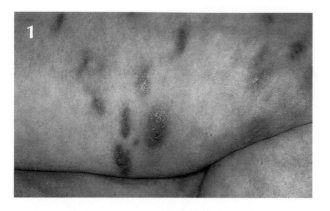

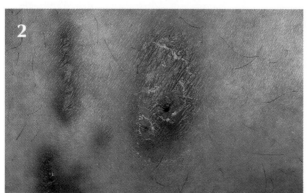

MYCOBACTERIUM CHELONAE MYCOBACTERIOSIS

In the case illustrated, the infection was due to mesotherapy (multiple subcutaneous microinstillation therapy) for cellulite. Purplish nodules, some in the process of abscess formation (Photo 1), appeared at each injection site in the weeks following. The distinctive feature of the nodules is their oblong shape (Photo 2) caused by the fact that the injections were so close together as to be almost contiguous.

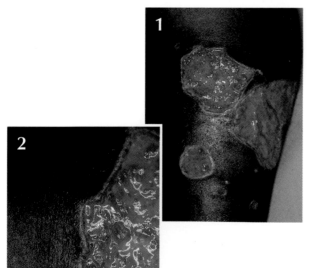

TROPICAL MYCOBACTERIUM ULCERANS MYCOBACTERIOSIS : BURULI ULCER

Buruli ulcer is purely tropical, being found in central Africa, Australia, New Guinea, and the north east of South America. It is due to *Mycobacterium ulcerans* and is aquatic in origin (marshes, rivers, lakes), favored by grazes on the legs. It is non contagious. The lesions are multiple ulcerations (Photo 1), often with little or no systemic impact. They grow inexorably and have a slightly raised border (Photo 2).

LEISHMANIASIS

Cutaneous leishmaniasis, which is worldwide though confined to particular regions, is caused by *Leishmania spp.* Though primarily confined to the indigenous population of endemic regions, it is a well-recognized imported dermatosis, presenting at skin clinics worldwide as it can readily be contracted during trips abroad. Though intercontinental tourism is the major culprit, occupational factors also play a role, e.g. business trips, foreign aid programs, managerial functions at construction sites etc.

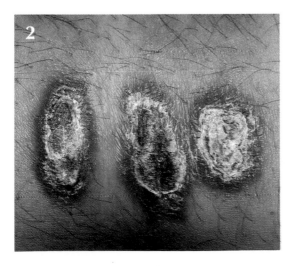

L. TROPICA OLD WORLD AND MEDITERRANEAN BASIN (MIDDLE EAST) LEISHMANIASIS

After 2–3 months incubation, a purplish erythematous nodule (Photo 1) appears with a central ulcer, the base of which consists of serum, blood and pus. The lesion is painless and slow-growing. The patient in this case was a foreign aid worker stationed 50 kilometers from Aleppo ("Aleppo boil"). Another foreign aid worker in the same area presented with three oblong nodules which are purplish, keratotic and painless (Photo 2).

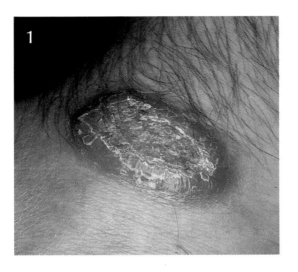

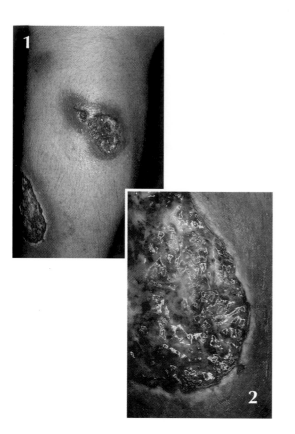

L. GUYANENSIS AMERICAN LEISHMANIASIS (SOUTH AND CENTRAL AMERICA)

Crusting ulcers with a mildly keratotic rim (Photo 1) due to *Leishmania guyanensis*. Painless, slow-growing and non inflammatory, they resolve spontaneously after several months or years leaving a permanent scar. Some ulcers are several centimeters in diameter (Photo 2), with some granulation tissue in their erythematous or fibrinous base. They are surrounded by a thin flat purplish ring (unlike the lesions due to *Pyoderma gangrenosum*). This patient was a Belgian researcher on a survival experiment in the Guyana forest, along the banks of the River Maroni.

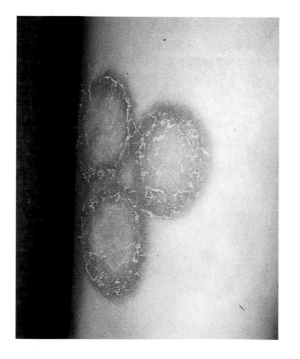

TINEA CORPORIS

Three perfectly circular erythemato-squamous lesions of recent onset, in the process of gradual excentric spread. The centre of each lesion is the same color as the normal skin, with few squames: spontaneous regression is underway. Direct microscopy of the squames showed dermatophyte filaments, identified as *Microsporum* canis on culture. The history included recent contact with a contaminated cat.

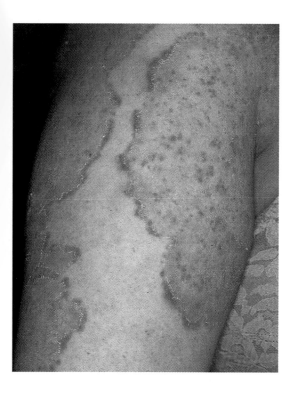

EXTENSIVE TINEA CORPORIS IN IMMUNODEPRESSED SUBJECTS

Extensive sharply marginated erythemato-squamous plaques with low-grade infiltration. The plaque centres are scattered with erythematous and occasionally vesicular minipapules. Direct microscopy of the squames showed dermatophyte filaments, identified as *Trichophyton rubrum* on culture. Without appropriate therapy, the infection has no tendency to resolve; in the case illustrated the subject had impaired cell-mediated immunity. Repeated topical steroid application would probably cause an identical picture.

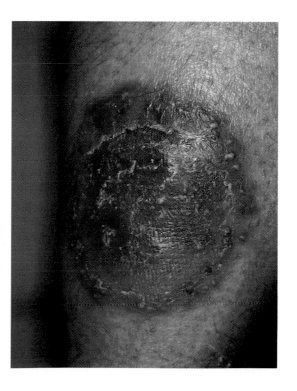

DERMATOPHYTOSIS WITH A FOLLICULITIS COMPONENT

Large, round, infiltrated erythemato-squamous plaque dotted with multiple follicular pustules on the extensor aspect of the leg in a farmer's wife, simultaneously with an epidemic of bovine ringworm in her cattle.
Direct microscopy of the squames and follicular pus showed dermatophyte filaments and spores, identified as *Trichophyton verrucosum* on culture.

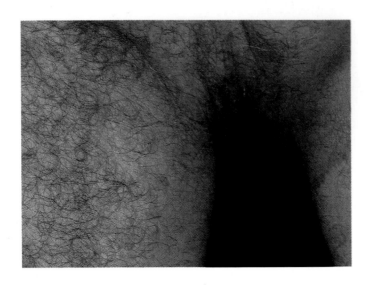

TINEA CRURIS

Sharply marginated and slightly infiltrated erythemato-squamous plaque in the groin.

Tinea cruris is commoner in men than in women, and is often combined with *tinea pedis*. Direct microscopy of the squames showed dermatophyte filaments, identified in this largely non inflammatory lesion as *Trichophyton rubrum*.

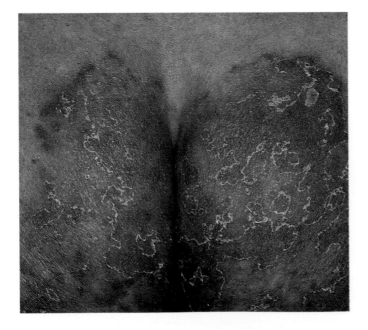

TINEA GLUTEALIS

Extensive infiltrated erythemato-squamous plaque on both buttocks. The sharply marginated border is vesicular in places. Buttock involvement is usually associated with *tinea cruris* and/or *tinea pedis*. Culture of this highly inflammatory lesion identified *Trichophyton interdigitale*.

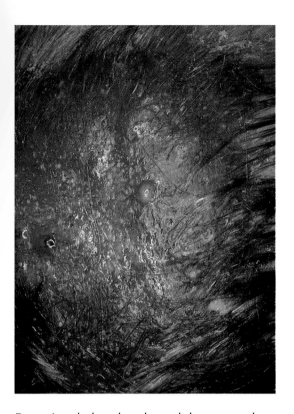

KERION CELSI

By definition kerion celsi is an inflammatory prominent nodule of sudden onset which grows rapidly (up to several centimeters in diameter) and is of tumor-like appearance.

From the occupational standpoint, it is usually due to *Trichophyton verrucosum*, a zoophilic dermatophyte which usually parasitizes cattle. It is thus largely found in rural areas.

Extensive dark-red scalp nodule scattered with follicular pustules. The infected hairs have totally disappeared. Residual cicatricial alopecia persists after cure.

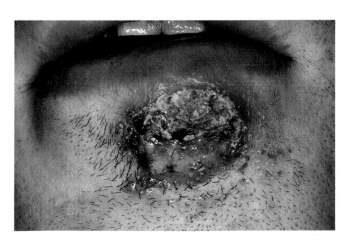

Nodular, crusting exudative lesion of the chin, with complete hair loss.

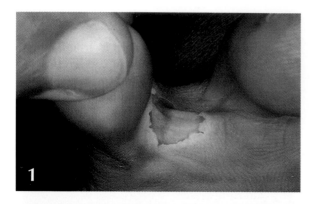

TINEA PEDIS

Widely known as athlete's foot. Lesions tend to be squamous and fissured. The most common site is the 4th interdigital web, particularly in the presence of hyperhidrosis, as in wearers of occlusive footwear. Infection is contracted in swimming pools, municipal baths, and from the carpeting of public buildings.

The most common dermatophyte pathogens are *Trichophyton interdigitale, Trichophyton rubrum, Trichophyton mentagrophytes,* and *Epidermophyton floccosum.*

Photo 1.
Whitish diffuse maceration in the cleft marginated by a collarette of continuous desquamation.

Photo 2.
A small painful fissure running along the line of the cleft. The entire area is ulcerative and macerated from microbial superinfection.

Photo 3.
Tinea pedis is sometimes associated with reactive plantar pompholyx: extremely pruritic coalescent vesicular eczema.

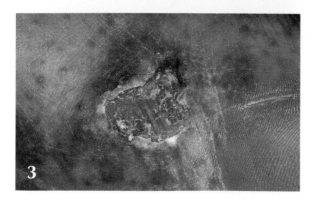

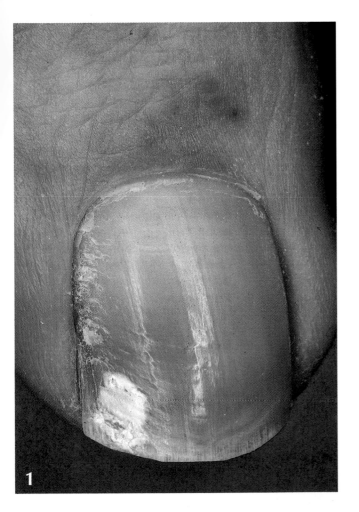

DERMATOPHYTE ONYCHOMYCOSIS

A frequent condition which may be isolated or associated with mycosis of the surrounding skin: *tinea pedis, tinea manuum* etc. It affects one or more toenails; it is less common on the hands. The infection begins at the distal extremity of the nail bed or nail fold.

Photo 1.
Onychomycosis with leukonychia affecting part of the distal nail extremity but also extending along a nail fold towards the cuticle. Full-thickness destruction of the nail, including the superficial plate, accounts for the pearly mat appearance of the infected area.

Photo 2.
Massive destruction of the nail, spicules of which have become detached all along the free border. The irregular pigmentation – whitish at some points and bright yellow at others – suggests mixed infection with dermatophytes and opportunistic yeasts (*Scopulariopsis brevicaulis*).

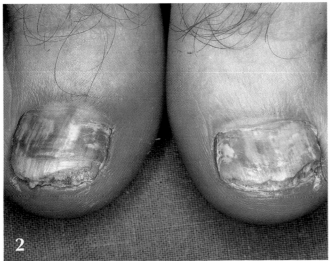

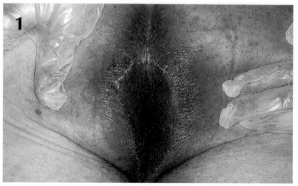

CUTANEOUS CANDIDIASIS

The pathogen belongs to the yeast-like fungal species, Candida. These fungi are dimorphic (with yeast and mycelian forms).
Candidiasis mainly affects the skin folds, particularly when macerated.

Photo 1.
Perianal candidiasis. Erythematous lesion, with erosion and a peripheral ring of desquamation. In the present case it was associated with gastrointestinal candidiasis (following destruction of the microflora ecosystem by antibiotic therapy).

Photo 2.
Candidiasis of the submammary fold. Glazed open plaque along the fold line. Note the collarettes of desquamation and the margins of multiple characteristic punctate papular pustules. Contributory factors include obesity and diabetes.

Photo 3.
Interdigital *Candida intertrigo* and *Candida paronychia* in a baker.
The contributory factor was repeated contact with detergents and sugars.

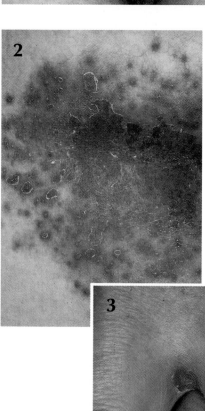

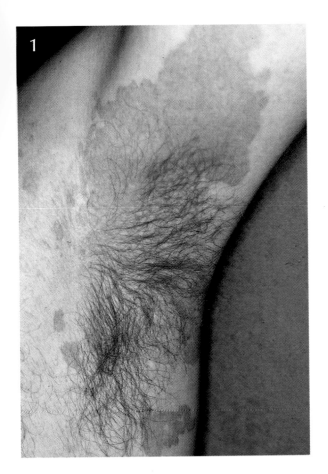

PITYRIASIS VERSICOLOR

A cosmopolitan dermatosis caused by a lipophilic yeast which is part of the skin flora, *Pityrosporum ovale* (or *orbiculare*), in its mycelian phase, *Malassezia furfur*.

Climatic heat and humidity encourage its appearance and/or spread in tropical countries. In temperate climates, it becomes more common in summer, particularly in athletes.

Photo 1.
Vast and slightly squamous fawn-yellow plaque with a distinct polycyclic margin. As in most cases, the deep axillary fold is unaffected.

Photo 2.
Minimal scaling can be emphasized by scraping the skin with a scalpel.

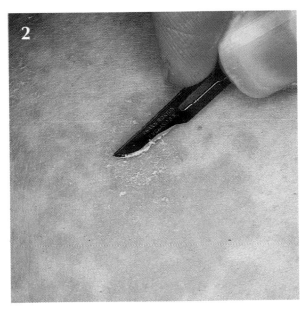

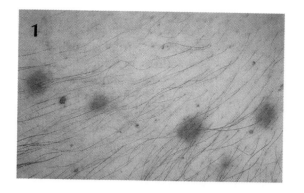

ARTHROPOD BITES

Insect bite lesions are polymorphous in appearance: they may be erythemato-papular, bullous, or occasionally purpuric. The variety in clinical appearance is probably due to a combination of two factors: the substance injected, and the subject's immune response.

The linear or bunched pattern of the lesions points to the diagnosis.

Photo 1.
Linearly distributed papulo-erythematous lesions. The bite is marked by a central punctate erosion in one lesion.

Photo 2.
Erythematous vesiculo-bullous lesions. This appearance is particularly common on the lower limbs.

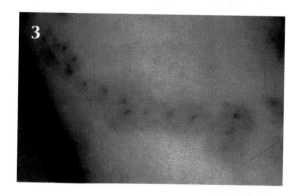

Photo 3.
Fleabites. The lesions are typical in distribution, number and convergence of the surrounding erythematous inflammatory reactions.

Photo 4.
Harvest mite bites (cutaneous trombiculosis). The purpuric erythemato-papular lesions give way to transient brownish macules. The lesions are concentrated in the skin folds and points of friction with clothes.

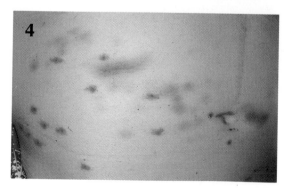

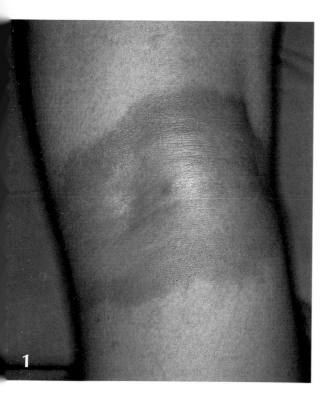

BORRELIOSIS : COMPLICATIONS OF TICK BITES

Tick bites can cause Borrelia infection. The cutaneous manifestations include *erythema migrans*, lymphocytoma and (Pick-Herxheimer) chronic atrophic acrodermatitis.

Photo 1.
Erythema migrans (Lyme disease). Extensive centrifugal erythema with a zone of clearing behind the advancing ring. Lyme disease refers only to New World borreliosis; it is improper for European borreliosis.

Photo 2.
Benign cutaneous lymphocytoma. Dark-red puffy nodule on the ridge of the nose.

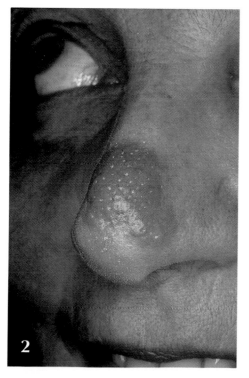

LARVA MIGRANS

The pathogen is an Ancylostoma larva which migrates at an approximate rate of 1 cm/day.

The characteristic feature of the lesion is an inflamed wandering track ending in a small papule marking the position of the larva.

Humans usually contract the infection on tropical beaches (contaminated by animal feces), i.e. it is an imported, non occupational dermatosis which tends to present on return from vacation.

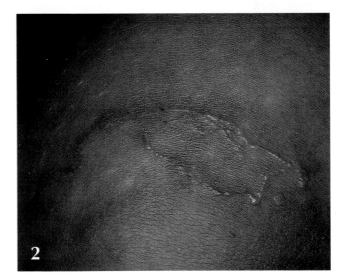

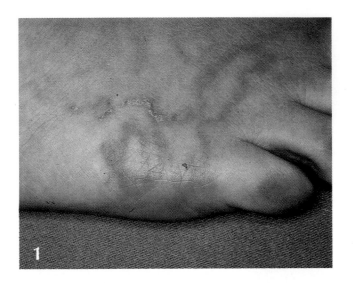

Photo 1.
Larva migrans in the foot, contracted in central Africa.

Photo 2.
Larva migrans of the breast, following a visit to Guadeloupe.

X. PSYCHODERMATOSES

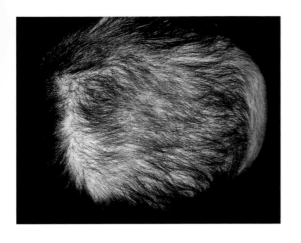

TRICHOTILLOMANIA

Hair-pulling habit tic causing non cicatricial circumscribed alopecia, often
either side of the midline. In this case
the area of alopecia is rectangular and
shows broken hairs of irregular length.

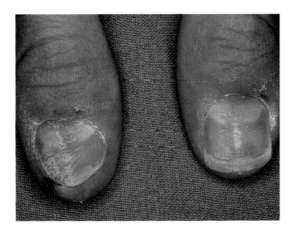

ONYCHOTILLOMANIA

Nailfold-tearing habit tic, resulting in
hangnails (hard pieces of epidermis
breaking away from the lateral nail
folds).
The multiple small horizontal furrows of
the mid part of the nail plate, associated
with vertical depression along the entire
nail length, are due to another habit tic
– repeated friction from another nail of
the hand.

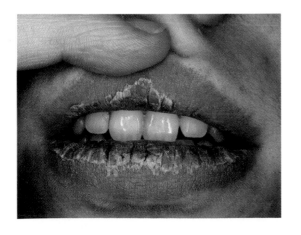

EXFOLIATIVE
(FACTITIOUS) CHEILITIS

Lip tic – involving repeated sucking and
chewing – has caused keratotic fissured
cheilitis of the vermilion (Klein's area)
along the whole length of the lower lip.

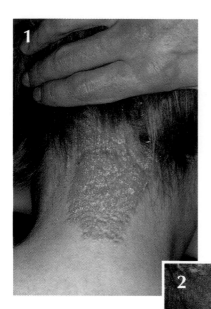

LICHENIFICATION (CIRCUMSCRIBED NEURODERMATITIS)

Dark-red or brown tree bark thickening of the skin caused by scratching but which itself then becomes a source of pruritus. Lichenification may be primary, or secondary to a dermatosis, e.g. eczema.

Photos 1 & 2.
Lichenification of the nape of the neck. Rectangular erythemato-squamous plaque (Photo 1) invading the scalp. The skin is scored by exaggerated normal markings. Detached scales vary in size (Photo 2).

Photo 3.
Perianal lichenification. Sharply marginated erythemato-squamous plaque showing multiple fissures and punctate erosions.

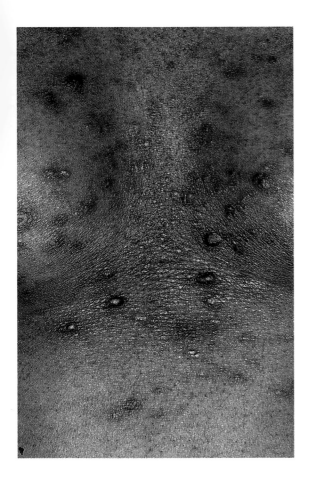

PRURIGO
(NEUROTIC EXCORIATION)

Prurigo is a widely used term in the dermatological literature but does not designate a clearly defined entity in clinical, histopathological or etiological terms.

Its main feature is an intensely pruritic and rapidly excoriated papular eruption. Prurigo may follow simple scratching with no underlying disease (as illustrated) or be associated with atopic dermatitis. It is also seen in AIDS.

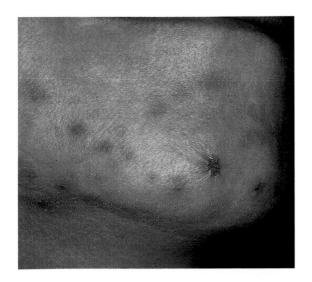

ACNE EXCORIÉE

Typical features of acne complicated by bleeding erosions due to repeated scratching, classically in girls. It is at any event more frequent in women than in men, and found mainly on the chin, though may also occur on the forehead, cheeks and neck. In the present case, the only acne lesions are a few papulo-pustules.

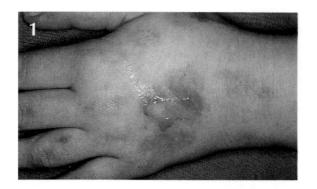

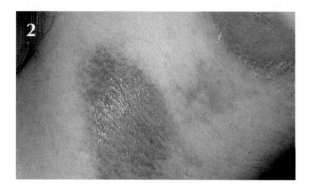

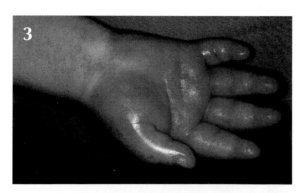

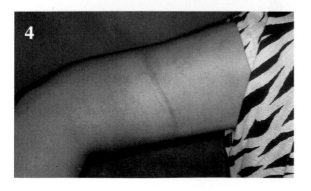

SIMULATED DERMATOSIS

This term covers all the pathological changes which individuals deliberately inflict on their skin and mucous membranes. True simulations are those caused by conscious subjects who deliberately mutilate themselves for illicit gain. Pathomimia, in the literal sense, is the mimicking of existing disease. In current usage, it refers solely to the lesions inflicted by psychologically disturbed individuals who simulate with relative unawareness, with no apparent motive for illicit gain.

Photo 1.
Simulated dermatosis on the back of the hand in a young woman using a caustic agent to obtain sick leave. The lesion is erythemato-edematous with an ulcerated centre discharging abundant serum, blood and pus.

Photo 2.
Dermatitis artefacta on the lateral aspect of the neck in a severely disturbed woman. The lance-shaped lesions, which are self-inflicted, are erythematous, ulcerated, and sharply marginated.

Photos 3 & 4.
Secrétan syndrome, a variant of dermatitis artefacta, characterized by lymphedema of one or both hands (Photo 3), caused by wearing a constricting garment or band around the arm or forearm. The clue to diagnosis is an erythematous and perfectly regular horizontal ring around the limb proximal to the edema (Photo 4).

XI. HAND DERMATITIS AND ITS DIFFERENTIAL DIAGNOSIS

Hand dermatitis occupies a privileged place in environmental dermatology. In addition to classical contact dermatitis, there is a whole range of conditions, including psoriasis and Tinea manuum, which raise problems of differential diagnosis. This chapter is devoted to this diagnostic conundrum.

CONTACT IRRITANT DERMATITIS

Contact irritant dermatitis has a variety of clinical presentations in the hand depending on the area involved (dorsum, palm, digital pulp), the irritant concerned, its concentration, frequency of use etc.

For example :

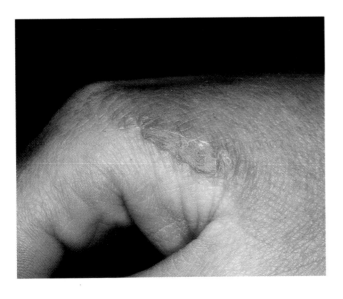

CONTACT IRRITANT DERMATITIS OF THE DORSUM OF THE HAND

Pruritic painful irritant dermatitis confined exclusively to the dorsum of the hand due to repeated contact with household detergents. Extensive, slightly squamous, erythematous plaque. Points of repeated wear-and-tear are thickened with pre-callus formation. There is a strikingly sharp divide between the irritated dorsal skin and intact palmar skin.

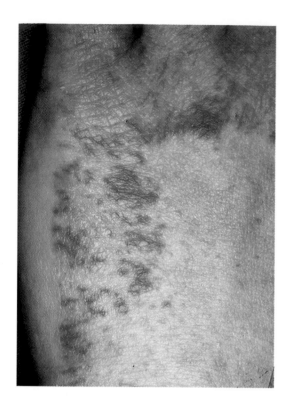

Irritant dermatitis of the dorsum of the hand in a female salon shampoo assistant. The lesions resemble eczema craquelé, with small parallel fissures; the topography mirrors the repeated flow of concentrated shampoo and is thus entirely occupational.

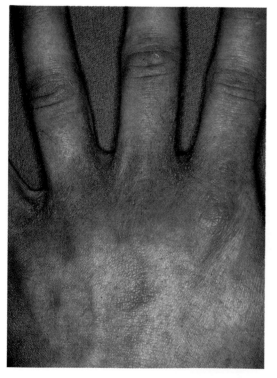

Chronic irritant dermatitis due to repeated maceration of the hands in brine (meat pickling worker). The erythemato-squamous lesions are concentrated on the skin overlying the metacarpo-phalangeal joints and in the interdigital clefts. There is associated pruritus, together with painful tugging sensations.

CONTACT IRRITANT DERMATITIS OF THE PALM OF THE HAND

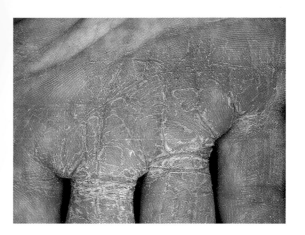

Large sharply marginated erythemato-squamous plaque in a butcher due to repeated contact with wet meat, hence the occupationally determined topography.

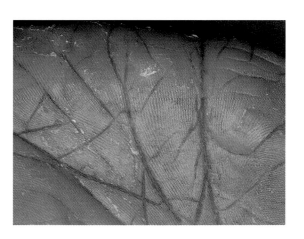

Chronic irritant dermatitis showing peeling on a diffuse erythematous background. The natural skin folds are accentuated, as if hollowed out, and encrusted with blackish dust-like debris. This used to be termed "housewive's dermatitis" and is characteristic of repeated friction on the palm, usually in a wet environment (window cleaner, in the case illustrated).

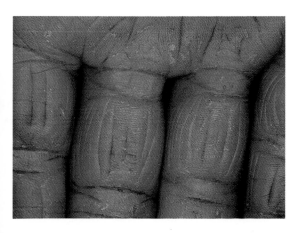

Chronic irritant dermatitis affecting the palmar aspect of the fingers. Faint and sometimes even absent fingerprints on a diffuse erythemato-squamous background (wear-and-tear dermatitis). Conversely, the natural skin folds are accentuated and encrusted with dirt. This patient is a machine tool assembly plant worker in permanent contact with soluble oil.

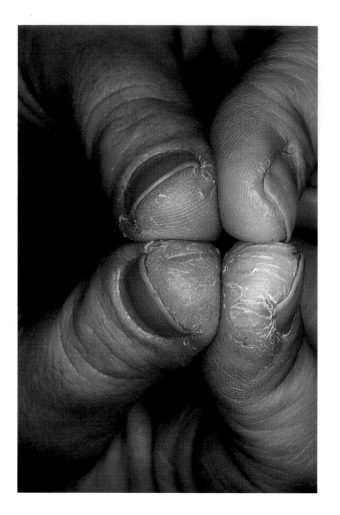

IRRITANT DERMATITIS: FINGERTIP DERMATITIS

Occupational fissured acropulpitis of the right thumb and index finger in a female post office worker due to repeated friction with a wet pad (sticking stamps). The fingerprints have disappeared. The fissures and bands of desquamation follow a linear distribution. They cause permanent and sometimes painful discomfort.

ALLERGIC CONTACT DERMATITIS

Allergic contact dermatitis of the hand has a variety of clinical presentations ranging from the extremely acute to the extremely chronic. The topography is informed by the nature of the contact with the chemical agent responsible.

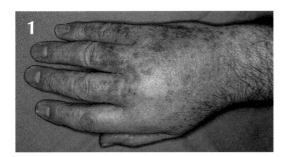

ALLERGIC CONTACT DERMATITIS OF THE DORSUM OF THE HAND AND/OR FINGERS

Photos 1 & 2.
Acute erythemato-vesicular allergic contact dermatitis on the dorsa of the hands and fingers in a roofer. The wood tar patch test was strongly positive. The topography is occupational determined.

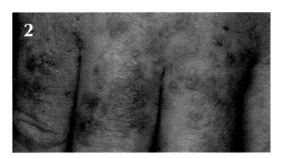

Photos 3 & 4.
Acute, erosive and crusting allergic contact dermatitis of the fingertips due to epoxy resins in a DIY enthusiast. The lesion topography, confined strictly to the fingers, emphasizes the precision of the movements involved. The fingernails are intact, thus marking the eczema as acute. The epoxy resin patch test was positive.

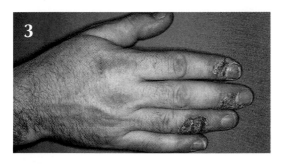

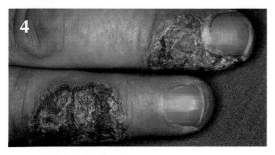

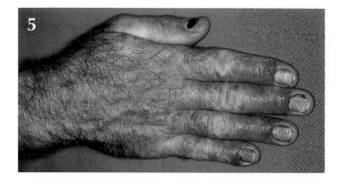

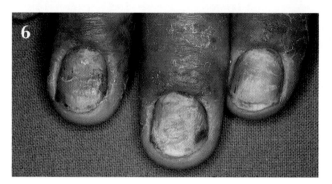

Photos 5 & 6.
Allergic contact dermatitis to cement chromate in a bricklayer. The dorsal tips of the fingers show erythema and erosion; the nail folds are edematous. The nail plates are affected: their surface is rough and friable. Nail involvement marks the eczema as chronic, with recurrent acute-on-chronic episodes timed by bouts of intensive work. The potassium dichromate patch test was positive.

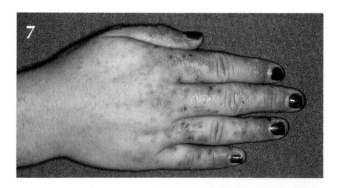

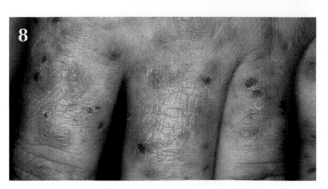

Photos 7 & 8.
Chronic allergic contact dermatitis of the dorsa of the hands and fingers in a female hairdresser, symptomatic of allergy to para-phenylenediamine (PPD), an ingredient of hair dyes. The lesions are slightly erythematous and highly pruritic, hence the multiple erosions. The fact that the lesions are confined to the distal dorsa of the hands is explained by the precision of the occupational movement involved. The PPD patch test was positive.

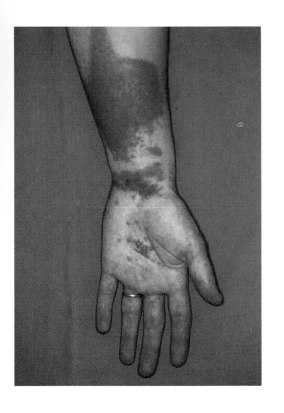

PALMAR ALLERGIC CONTACT DERMATITIS

Acute allergic contact dermatitis of the right palm and flexor aspect of the right forearm in a physiotherapist. The allergen was ketoprofen, used as an antiinflammatory for massaging painful joints in sports medicine. There is extensive forearm erythema, while the palm is dotted with tense vesicles converging into small bullae, mimicking acute pompholyx. The ketoprofen patch test was positive.

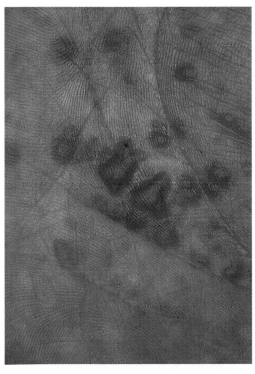

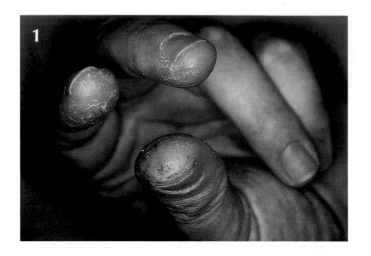

ALLERGIC CONTACT FINGER DERMATITIS

Photo 1.
Fissured acropulpitis of the right thumb, index and middle fingers from handling tulip bulbs. This is a case of allergic contact pulpitis, to be differentiated from simple irritation pulpitis. Patch tests with a bulb sliver and tuliposide A were both positive.

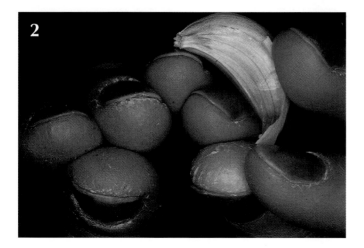

Photo 2.
Allergic contact acropulpitis in a female cook handling cloves of garlic. In this case the eczema consists solely of shallow fissures more reminiscent of contact irritant pulpitis. However the diagnosis of allergic contact dermatitis was given by the positive patch tests to the garlic allergens, diallyldisulfide and allicin.

Photo 3.
Allergic contact pulpitis involving the entire thumb in a dentist. The lesions are erythemato-squamous; the skin is edematous. Patch tests to the various acrylates and methacrylates used in dental fillings were positive.

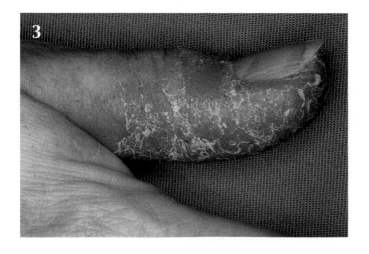

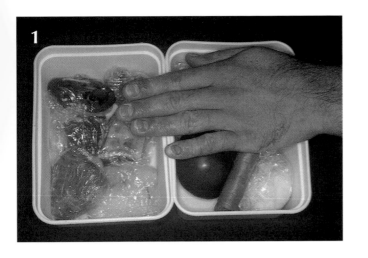

PROTEIN IMMUNE CONTACT DERMATITIS

Photo 1.
Various animal and vegetable proteins can penetrate the skin and cause contact dermatitis via an immune mechanism involving IgE. This is a case of protein dermatitis on the dorsal aspect of the fingers in a cook who supplied the main foods he handled at work for prick tests.

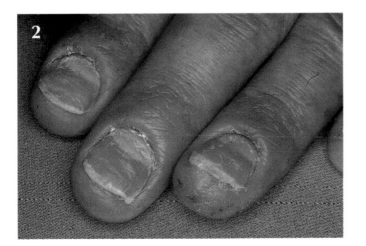

Photo 2.
Typical clinical presentation of protein immune contact dermatitis, showing striking paronychia and nail changes consisting of irregular striae of the plate associated with yellowish onycholysis. The prick test to a sample of monkfish was strongly positive. The diagnosis provided a basis for redistributing labor within the restaurant kitchen.

POMPHOLYX

This is an endogenous eczema of the palms and lateral aspects of the fingers which is not due to contact allergens but is exacerbated by contact with irritants, especially in warm and humid environments. It is seen mainly but not exclusively in young women. Patch tests do not usually aid diagnosis, but if positive they can justify oral challenge tests which can exacerbate the lesions in some subjects (especially in the case of nickel and balsam of Peru). Pompholyx may also be plantar, involving the lateral aspects of the toes, and may be found in association with *tinea pedis*, in what has been termed pompholyx dermatophytide.

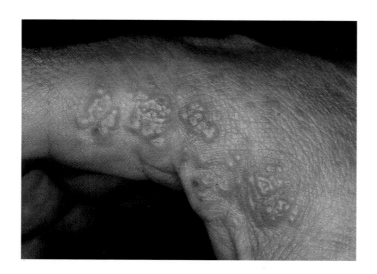

VESICULAR POMPHOLYX OF THE LATERAL ASPECTS OF THE FINGERS

The pompholyx vesicles are bunched on the lateral aspects of the fingers. They are hard to the touch, embedded in epidermis, and translucent. They are associated with intense pruritus.

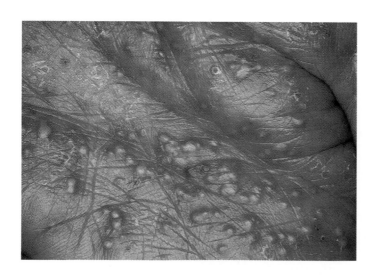

VESICULAR PALMAR POMPHOLYX

Isolated and confluent pompholyx vesicles are scattered over the palm. Incipient pustulization is present. There is intense pruritus.

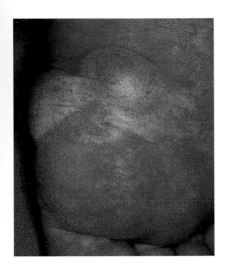

BULLOUS PLANTAR POMPHOLYX

The pompholyx vesicles embedded in plantar epidermis have converged into large painful bullae. In the present case, the pompholyx episode occurred at the end of a long summer walk. It is idiopathic, in that it is not associated with *tinea pedis*.

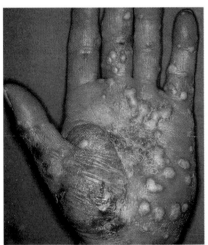

PALMAR PUSTULAR POMPHOLYX

Pompholyx vesiculo-bullae have transformed into tense pustules scattered over the entire palm and palmar aspect of the fingers.

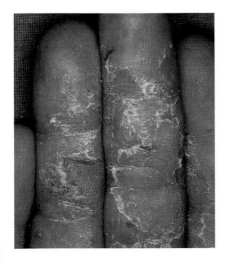

DESQUAMATORY REGRESSIVE POMPHOLYX

Pompholyx of the palmar and lateral aspects of the fingers in a female textile worker whose hands spend several hours a day in a soluble oil. The lesions regressed gradually over several days off work. The receding lesions are eczematous and erythemato-squamous.

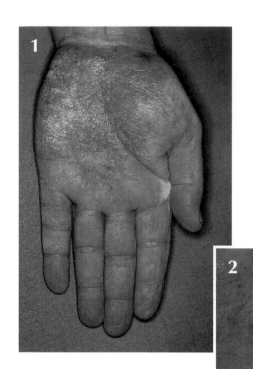

PALMAR POMPHOLYX ECZEMA

The palm shows extensive, dry, highly pruritic erythemato-squamous eczema (Photo 1). High magnification (Photo 2) shows multiple vesicles, some of which have burst, dotted over the entire eczema surface.

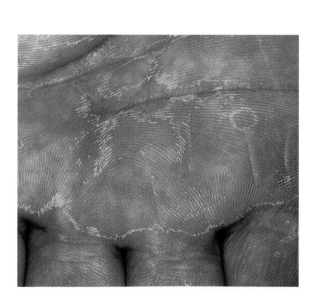

RECURRENT FOCAL PALMAR PEELING (DESQUAMATION ESTIVALE EN AIRES DES MAINS)

This highly distinctive condition occurs only in summer, disappearing (sometimes incompletely) in winter. It is unrelated to external irritation. It affects the palmar aspect of the hands and fingers, and simply consists of dry and extremely superficial detachment of the epidermis. Initially, and in mild cases, the lesion is the size of a small pinhead. It then broadens slightly with a small circular but soon incomplete border. Peeling often spreads excentrically and the various circles may converge in wavy lines.

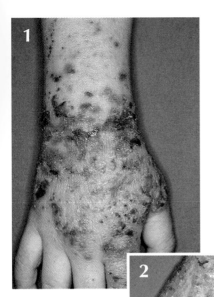

ATOPIC DERMATITIS OF THE HANDS

Atopic subjects with or without evidence of atopic dermatitis in other body areas may develop hand eczema from contact irritants. The cardinal features are intense pruritus, a predilection for the dorsum of the hands and fingers, and a random distribution, i.e. avoiding some areas but in a manner that differs from patient to patient, as shown in the following illustrations.

Photo 1.
Acute exudative eczema with yellowish crusts and scratch marks. Massive staphylococcal colonization. Note the involvement of the dorsum of the index finger; absolutely no other fingers are involved.

Photo 2.
Chronic, crusting, deeply-fissured eczema. The dorsa of the hand, thumb, index and middle fingers are entirely covered in eczema, while the ring and little finger are unaffected.

Photo 3.
Chronic erythemato-squamous eczema with erosions and fissures, spreading symmetrically to the dorsa of all the fingers and distal dorsa of the hands, while leaving the proximal parts intact. The topography is highly characteristic of atopic dermatitis.

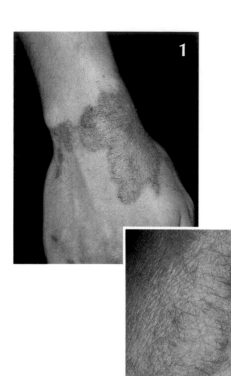

NUMMULAR ECZEMA OF THE DORSA OF THE HANDS

This form of eczema is characterized by single or multiple round or oval erythematous plaques, which may be isolated or confluent (Photo 1). Higher magnification (Photo 2) shows vesicles on the plaque margins. Nummular eczema is endogenous in origin but exacerbated in a humid environment.

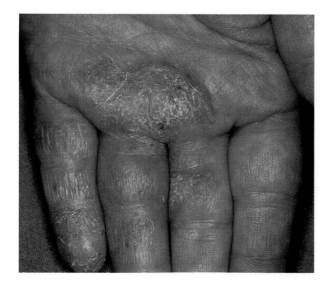

PALMAR NUMMULAR ECZEMA

Nummular eczema obeys a distinctive topography on the palm, involving the flexor aspect of the fingers and fanning in a semi-circle over the metacarpophalangeal joints, in a pattern resembling an apron (apron eczema). In the case illustrated, the eczema is dry and erythemato-squamous.

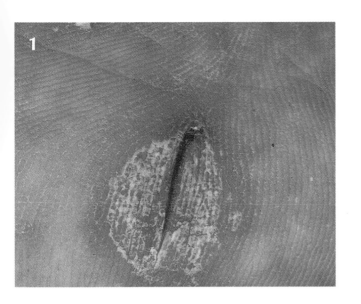

HYPERKERATOTIC PALMAR ECZEMA

Clinical presentations vary and probably encompass different entities produced by a combination of endogenous and mechanically repetitive exogenous factors. It is thus seen in conjunction with manual work, as an occupational or leisure activity condition. In some cases, the differential diagnosis with palmar psoriasis can be difficult. The presence of psoriasis elsewhere on the body may help to clarify the situation in some cases.

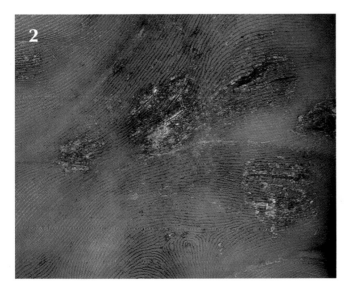

Photo 1.
The basic lesion of hyperkeratotic palmar eczema. A well-demarcated erythemato-squamous plaque is traversed by a deep fissure due to the absence of cutaneous elasticity on skin traction during manual work.

Photo 2.
Multiple hyperkeratotic dirt-encrusted lesions of the palm with scattered fissures. The near-nodular lesions constitute true callosities. In this particular case mechanical factors and repeated microtrauma played a predominant role.

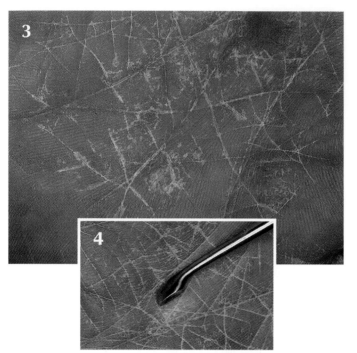

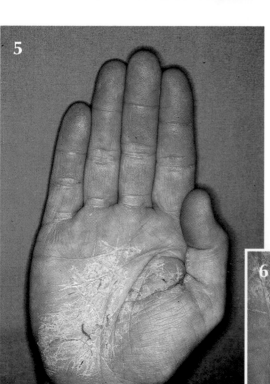

Photos 3 & 4.
Very mild variant of hyper-keratotic palmar eczema, featuring squamous accentuation of the natural skin folds (Photo 3). Scraping yields no squamous material, as the scales are highly adherent. This preliminary manoeuvre provides the differential diagnosis from *Tinea manuum*, in which scraping yields abundant squamous material.

Photos 5 & 6.
The most classic variant of hyperkeratotic palmar eczema, showing an extensive non erythematous squamous plaque with scattered fissures. It is this variant which is most difficult to differentiate from palmar psoriasis. In the present case there was no psoriasis elsewhere on the body nor any history of psoriasis.

PALMAR AND UNGUAL PSORIASIS

Palmar psoriasis is either isolated or associated with plantar psoriasis (palmoplantar psoriasis). It is also associated in some cases with characteristic nail lesions. The lesions are exacerbated by mechanical factors or microtrauma (Köbner phenomenon) and are thus produced by a combination of endogenous and exogenous factors.

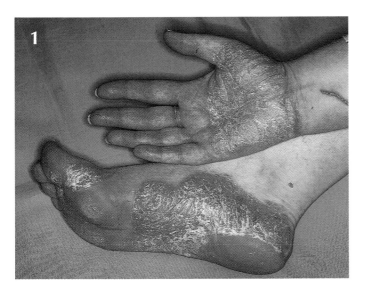

PALMOPLANTAR PSORIASIS

Perfectly delimited erythemato-squamous lesions. Two points should be noted: first, the lesions have spread to the mediolateral aspect of the foot, which confirms standard descriptions (Photo 1); second, the psoriasis is confined strictly to the palm, without invading the flexor aspect of the forearm, as if the limits of the lesions had been drawn strictly to plan (Photo 2).

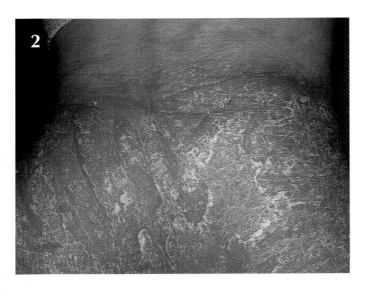

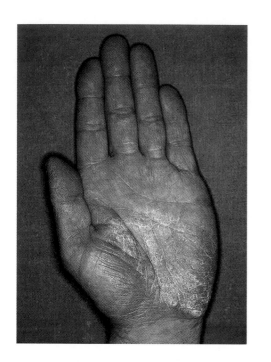

ISOLATED PALMAR PSORIASIS

Keratotic erythemato-squamous plaque strictly within the confines of the palm. The lesion in no way differs from hyperkeratotic palmar dermatitis except for the surrounding zone of erythema. Only the history and clinical examination of the rest of the skin point to one or other diagnosis.

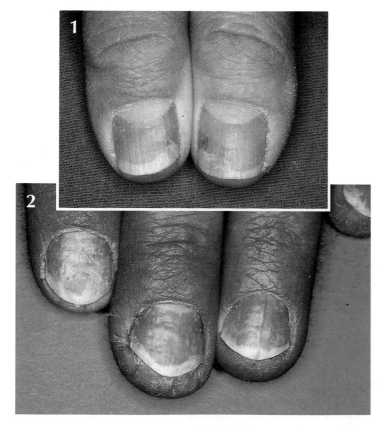

NAIL INVOLVEMENT IN PSORIASIS

Photo 1.
Two classic signs of nail involvement in psoriasis are clearly recognizable: distal onycholysis and filiform hematomata. Exacerbation by mechanical factors (Köbner phenomenon) is obvious.

Photo 2.
The classic image of nail involvement in psoriasis. Erythemato-squamous psoriasis of the finger tip. The nail signs are distal onycholysis and multiple punctate thimble-shaped depressions.

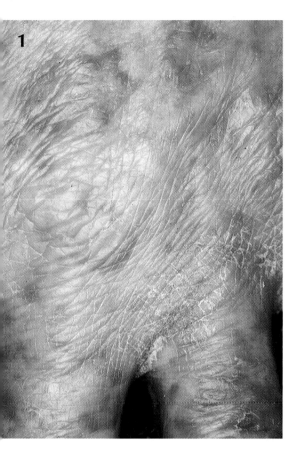

TINEA MANUUM

Tinea manuum is a diagnostic trap with regard to chronic eczema. In most cases it is strictly unilateral, which provides a first clue to the diagnosis. It may or may not be associated with other dermatophyte lesions: *tinea pedis, tinea cruris*. It can be isolated and may be precipitated by gardening or other activity involving contact with contaminated soil (geophilic dermatophyte).

Photo 1.
Tinea manuum of the dorsum of the hand, characterized by small, round, well-delimited erythemato-squamous lesions. In the present case, application of a topical corticosteroid reduced the inflammatory component of the lesions and resulted in the appearance of small pustules along the lesion edges.

Photo 2.
Tinea manuum of the interdigital webs and dorsa of the fingers. Squamous erythema over the fingers with pearl white accentuation of desquamation in the natural folds of the interdigital clefts.

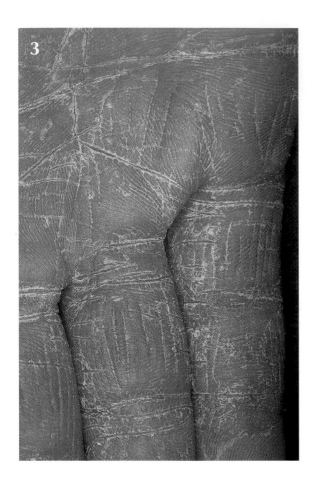

Photo 3.
Tinea manuum of the palm and palmar aspect of the fingers. Dusty desquamation on an erythematous background with pearl white accentuation of the palmar flexor folds. The appearance is very similar to that of some cases of hyperkeratotic palmar eczema, but in *Tinea manuum*, scraping yields a flurry of disintegrating scales.

Photo 4.
Palmar *Tinea manuum* scrapings yielding a harvest of floury scales which, after cleaning with potassium hydroxide, were shown on direct microscopy to contain concentrated dermatophyte filaments.

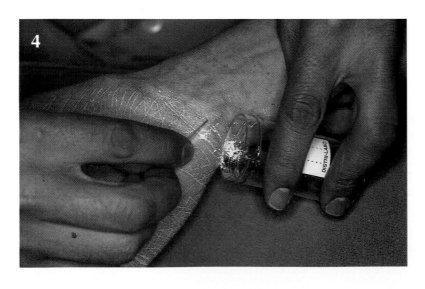

XII. SKIN TEST TECHNIQUES

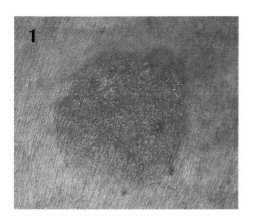

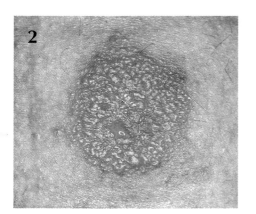

PATCH TESTS

The etiological diagnosis of allergic contact dermatitis involves allergen identification using standardized patch test techniques. Patches are applied for 48 hours; results are read twice, first at 48 hours, then at 96 hours (failing which, a single reading is performed at 72 hours). Positive tests are read in compliance with International Contact Dermatitis Research Group (ICDRG) recommendations.

Photo 1.
Patch test ++: erythema, infiltration, papules, a few vesicles. Read at 72 hours.

Photo 2.
Patch test ++: erythema, infiltration, confluent crop of vesicles. Read at 48 hours.

Photo 3.
Patch test +++: erythema, major infiltration, coalescent vesicles forming a bulla. Read at 48 hours.

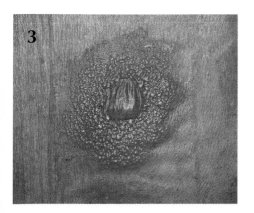

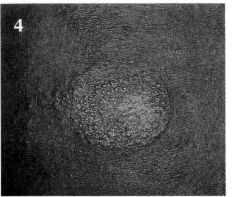

Photo 4.
Patch test ++: on a black skin, darkening of the skin color replaces erythema. Infiltration and vesicles. Read at 72 hours.

Photo 5.
Patch test ++: the skin appears dark, major infiltration of the central part, whitish tense vesicles mimicking minipustules. This particular image is due to the greater thickness of the stratum corneum in Blacks. The vesicles only burst as tension increases. Read at 48 hours.

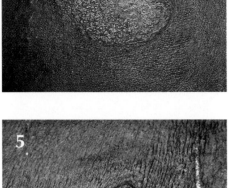

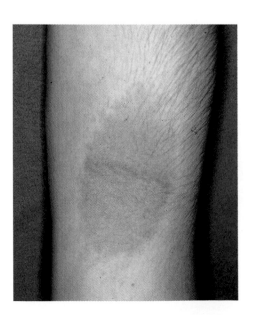

REPEATED OPEN APPLICATION TEST (ROAT)

The ROAT can be a useful complement to patch tests, in particular where cosmetics are involved. The finished product (perfume, lotion, cream etc) is applied twice daily to a specific skin area (flexor aspect of the forearm or antecubital fossa). Application is stopped if the result is positive. If negative after 14 successive applications, the test is stopped.
The figure shows a positive test with an eau de toilette.

INDEX